Key Consultations in Hepatology

Guest Editor

PAUL MARTIN, MD

CLINICS IN LIVER DISEASE

www.liver.theclinics.com

Consulting Editor
NORMAN GITLIN, MD

May 2009 • Volume 13 • Number 2

SAUNDERS an imprint of ELSEVIER, Inc.

W.B. SAUNDERS COMPANY

A Division of Elsevier Inc.

1600 John F. Kennedy Boulevard, Suite 1800 • Philadelphia, PA 19103-2899

http://www.theclinics.com

CLINICS IN LIVER DISEASE Volume 13, Number 2
May 2009 ISSN 1089-3261, ISBN-13: 978-1-4377-0496-9, ISBN-10: 1-4377-0496-4

Editor: Kerry Holland
Developmental Editor: Donald Mumford

Clinics in Liver Disease (ISSN 1089-3261) is published quarterly by Elsevier Inc., 360 Park Avenue South, New York, NY 10010-1710. Months of issue are February, May, August, and November. Business and editorial offices: 1600 John F. Kennedy Boulevard, Suite 1800, Philadelphia, PA 19103-2899. Customer service office: 6277 Sea Harbor Drive, Orlando, FL 32887-4800. Periodicals postage paid at New York, NY, and additional mailing offices. Subscription prices are $218.00 per year (U.S. individuals), $109.00 per year (U.S. student/resident), $333.00 per year (U.S. institutions), $288.00 per year (foreign individuals), $151.00 per year (foreign student/resident), $401.00 per year (foreign instituitions), $251.00 per year (Canadian individuals), $151.00 per year (Canadian student/resident), and $401.00 per year (Canadian institutions). Foreign air speed delivery is included in all *Clinics* subscription prices. All prices are subject to change without notice. **POSTMASTER:** Send address changes to *Clinics in Liver Disease*, Elsevier Journals Customer Service, 11830 Westline Industrial Drive, St. Louis, MO 63146. **Customer Service (orders, claims, online, change of address): Elsevier Periodicals Customer Service, 11830 Westline Industrial Drive, St. Louis, MO 63146. Tel: 1-800-654-2452 (U.S. and Canada); 314-453-7041 (outside U.S. and Canada). Fax: 314-453-5170. E-mail: journalscustomerservice-usa@elsevier.com (for print support); journalsonlinesupport-usa@elsevier.com (for online support).**

Reprints. For copies of 100 or more of articles in this publication, please contact the Commercial Reprints Department, Elsevier Inc., 360 Park Avenue South, New York, NY 10010-1710. Tel.: 212-633-3812; Fax: 212-462-1935; E-mail: reprints@elsevier.com.

Clinics in Liver Disease is covered in *MEDLINE/PubMed (Index Medicus)*.

Printed and bound by CPI Group (UK) Ltd, Croydon, CR0 4YY

Transferred to Digital Print 2011

Contributors

GUEST EDITOR

PAUL MARTIN, MD
Professor of Medicine; Chief, Division of Hepatology, University of Miami Miller School of Medicine, Miami, Florida

AUTHORS

AIJAZ AHMED, MD
Associate Professor of Medicine, Division of Gastroenterology and Hepatology, Stanford University School of Medicine, Stanford, California

ASHUTOSH J. BARVE, MD, PhD
Assistant Professor, Division of Gastroenterology/Hepatology, Department of Medicine, University of Louisville School of Medicine, Louisville, Kentucky

KEITH FALKNER, PhD
Senior Research Associate, Division of Gastroenterology/Hepatology, Department of Medicine, University of Louisville School of Medicine, Louisville, Kentucky

LAWRENCE S. FRIEDMAN, MD
Professor, Department of Medicine, Harvard Medical School, Boston; Professor, Department of Medicine, Tufts University School of Medicine, Boston; Chair, Department of Medicine, Newton-Wellesley Hospital, Newton; Assistant Chief, Department of Medicine, Massachusetts General Hospital, Boston, Massachusetts

PRIYA GREWAL, MD
Assistant Professor of Medicine, Division of Liver Diseases, Recanati/Miller Transplantation Institute, The Mount Sinai Medical Center, New York, New York

MICHAEL KRIER, MD
Fellow, Division of Gastroenterology and Hepatology, Stanford University School of Medicine, Stanford, California

KAREN L. KROK, MD
Assistant Professor of Medicine, Division of Gastroenterology and Hepatology, University of Pennsylvania School of Medicine, Philadelphia, Pennsylvania

MICHAEL R. LUCEY, MD, FRCPI
Professor of Medicine; Chief, Section of Gastroenterology and Hepatology, University of Wisconsin School of Medicine and Public Health, Madison, Wisconsin

JORGE A. MARRERO, MD, MS
Keith S. Henley Medical Professor of Gastroenterology, Division of Gastroenterology, Department of Internal Medicine, University of Michigan, Ann Arbor, Michigan

PAUL MARTIN, MD
Professor of Medicine; Chief, Division of Hepatology, University of Miami Miller School of Medicine, Miami, Florida

CRAIG J. McCLAIN, MD
Professor, Departments of Medicine and Pharmacology and Toxicology; Associate Vice President for Translational Research; Distinguished University Scholar, University of Louisville School of Medicine; Louisville VAMC, Louisville, Kentucky

SANTIAGO J. MUNOZ, MD, FACP, FACG
Professor of Medicine, Temple School of Medicine; Director of Clinical Hepatology; Medical Director, Liver Transplant Program, Philadelphia, Pennsylvania

CAROLYN T. NGUYEN, BSN, MSN, CRNP
Division of Gastroenterology, Department of Medicine, Liver Transplant, Cedars-Sinai Medical Center, Los Angeles, California

CHRISTOPHER B. O'BRIEN, MD, FACG
Chief of Clinical Hepatology, Center for Liver Diseases; Professor of Clinical Medicine, Divisions of Liver and Gastrointestinal Transplantation, University of Miami Miller School of Medicine, Miami, Florida

JACQUELINE G. O'LEARY, MD, MPH
Division of Hepatology, Department of Internal Medicine, Baylor University Medical Center, Dallas, Texas

MIHIR PATEL, MD
Resident, Department of Medicine, University of Louisville School of Medicine, Louisville, Kentucky

AARON J. PUGH, DO
Resident, Department of Medicine, University of Louisville School of Medicine, Louisville, Kentucky

NILA RAFIQ, MD
Hepatology Fellow, Center for Liver Diseases at Inova Fairfax Hospital, Falls Church, Virginia

K. RAJENDER REDDY, MD
Professor of Medicine; Director of Hepatology; Medical Director for Liver Transplantation, Hospital of the University of Pennsylvania, Philadelphia, Pennsylvania

OREN SHAKED
Research Assistant, School of Medicine, Hospital of the University of Pennsylvania, Philadelphia, Pennsylvania

TRAM T. TRAN, MD
Associate Professor, Department of Medicine, Geffen UCLA School of Medicine; Medical Director, Liver Transplant, Cedars-Sinai Medical Center, Los Angeles, California

THEODORE WELLING, MD
Assistant Professor of Surgery, Division of Transplant, Department of Surgery, University of Michigan, Ann Arbor, Michigan

PATRICK S. YACHIMSKI, MD, MPH
Research Fellow, Department of Medicine, Harvard Medical School; Advanced Endoscopy Fellow, Gastrointestinal Unit, Massachusetts General Hospital; Division of Gastroenterology, Brigham and Women's Hospital, Boston, Massachusetts

ZOBAIR M. YOUNOSSI, MD, MPH
Professor of Medicine, Center for Integrated Research, Inova Health System, Falls Church, Virginia

Contents

> Traditionally, the constellation of biochemistry tests including liver enzymes, total bilirubin, and hepatic synthetic measures (prothrombin time (PT) and serum albumin level) are referred to as liver function tests (LFTs). Abnormal LFTs can be encountered during primary health care visits, routine blood donation, and insurance screening. A reported 1% to 4% of asymptomatic patients exhibit abnormal LFTs, leading to a sizeable number of annual consultations to a gastroenterology and/or hepatology practice. A cost-effective and systematic approach is essential to the interpretation of abnormal LFTs. A review of pattern of abnormal LFTs, detailed medical history, and a comprehensive physical examination help establish a foundation for further individualized testing. Further investigation often involves biochemical testing for disease-specific markers, radiographic imaging, and even consideration of a liver biopsy. In the following account, markers of hepatic injury are reviewed followed by a discussion on an approach to various patterns of abnormal LFTs in an asymptomatic patient.

> Evaluation of abnormal liver function tests (LFTs) in the hospitalized patient is typically more urgent than the outpatient setting. This process is best organized into four steps. The first step is to determine whether the abnormal LFTs are associated with the illness resulting in the admission to the hospital or preceded the present illness. The second is to determine the etiology of the underlying liver disease. The third step is to evaluate the severity of the liver dysfunction and determine if acute liver failure (ALF) or acute decompensation of chronic liver failure is present. The final step is to look for the presence of associated complications—either those of ALF or chronic liver failure as appropriate.

> Incidentally discovered liver masses are becoming more common with the increasing application and power of imaging techniques for the evaluation of abdominal conditions. Although such masses are often benign, conclusive diagnoses must be established in order to provide appropriate patient care. Various imaging modalities can be utilized to accurately diagnose such masses without resort to more invasive diagnostic measures.

cirrhosis. To treat alcoholic liver injury, corticosteroids have become the standard of care in patients with severe alcoholic hepatitis. In contrast, the role of pharmacotherapy to treat alcoholic fibrosis is unclear, with failure to observe a benefit in randomized, placebo-controlled clinical trials of colchicine, S-adenosylmethionine (SAMe), or phosphatidylcholine. Liver transplantation remains an option in selected patients with life-threatening alcoholic liver disease.

Drug-induced hepatotoxicity is underreported and underestimated in the United States. It is an important cause of acute liver failure. Common classes of drugs causing drug-induced hepatotoxicity include antibiotics, lipid lowering agents, oral hypoglycemics, psychotropics, antiretrovirals, acetaminophen, and complementary and alternative medications. Hepatotoxic drugs often have a signature or pattern of liver injury including patterns of liver test abnormalities, latency of symptom onset, presence or absence of immune hypersensitivity, and the course of the reaction after drug withdrawal.

The management of autoimmune and cholestatic liver disorders is a challenging area of hepatology. Autoimmune and cholestatic liver diseases represent a comparatively small proportion of hepatobiliary disorders, yet their appropriate management is of critical importance for patient survival. In this article, management strategies are discussed, including the indications and expectations of pharmacologic therapy, endoscopic approaches, and the role of liver transplantation.

The three most commonly identified causes of viral hepatitis in the United States are hepatitis A virus (HAV), hepatitis B virus (HBV), and hepatitis C virus (HCV). Hundreds of millions of people worldwide are infected by these viruses; many experience illness as a result. This article discusses current recommendations for vaccination and other forms of prophylaxis aimed at minimizing the clinical effects of these viruses.

Timely surveillance for varices and hepatocellular carcinoma, prophylaxis against spontaneous bacterial peritonitis (SBP) improve survival in patients awaiting transplantation. Early diagnosis of minimal or overt hepatic encephalopathy can delay life threatening complications, reduce need for hospitalization, and potentially improve survival pending liver transplantation.

FORTHCOMING ISSUES

August 2009
Novel Therapies in Hepatitis C Virus
Paul Pockros, MD, *Guest Editor*

November 2009
Non-Alcoholic Steatohepatitis
Stephen A. Harrison, MD, *Guest Editor*

RECENT ISSUES

February 2009
Coagulation and Hemostasis in Liver Disease: Controversies and Advances
Stephen H. Caldwell, MD, and
Arun J. Sanyal, MD, *Guest Editors*

November 2008
Hepatic Fibrosis: Pathogenesis, Diagnosis, and Emerging Therapies
Scott L. Friedman, MD, *Guest Editor*

August 2008
Hepatitis C Virus
K. Rajender Reddy, MD, and
David E. Kaplan, MD, MSc, *Guest Editors*

RELATED INTEREST

Gastroenterology Clinics of North America, June 2006, Vol. 35, No. 2
Common Gastrointestinal and Hepatic Infections
R. Goodgame, MD, and D.Y. Graham, MD, *Guest Editors*
http://www.gastro.theclinics.com/

THE CLINICS ARE NOW AVAILABLE ONLINE!

Access your subscription at:
www.theclinics.com

Preface

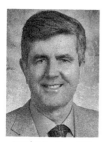

Paul Martin, MD
Guest Editor

A consequence of the rapid advances in the science and practice of hepatology has been an expanding number of diagnostic tests and therapeutic interventions. Although these new modalities have transformed the care of patients with liver disease, effective use of invasive, and often expensive, diagnostics is crucial.

In this issue of *Clinics in Liver Disease*, a group of distinguished hepatologists provide insight into the assessment of a variety of scenarios where clinical judgment based on experience and published literature is an invaluable addition to the care of individual patients. Assessment of hepatic dysfunction varies according to clinical circumstance—from the asymptomatic outpatient, as outlined by Drs. Krier and Ahmed, to the inpatient with severe medical illness, as described by Dr. O'Brien. Hepatic masses are frequently discovered during abdominal imaging, often for unrelated complaints, and require appropriate evaluation, as reviewed by Drs. Shaked and Reddy.

Preoperative clearance for surgery of a patient with underlying liver disease is important to assess perioperative risk and likelihood of postoperative hepatic decompensation, as outlined by Dr. Yachminski and coauthors. The increasing incidence and expanding treatment options for hepatocellular carcinoma has made management of this tumor a prominent part of current hepatology practice, as described by Drs. Welling and Marrero. The increasing prominence of nonalcoholic fatty liver disease is addressed by Drs. Rafiq and Younossi.

Although alcoholic liver disease continues to be a major challenge, there is renewed interest in its medical management, as well as appropriate indications for liver transplantation in abstinent patients, as reviewed by Dr. Lucey.

Dr. MacClain and colleagues address an issue of increasing concern, namely hepatotoxicity due to not only therapeutic agents but also herbal compounds. Newer immunosuppressants and other advances in the management of autoimmune and cholestatic liver diseases are reviewed by Drs. Krok and Munoz. An update on hepatitis vaccination is provided by Drs. Nguyen and Tran; and Dr. Grewal and I discuss the important role of the gastroenterologist and hepatologist in caring for the cirrhotic patient who may ultimately be bound for liver transplant.

Clin Liver Dis 13 (2009) xi–xii
doi:10.1016/j.cld.2009.04.001

liver.theclinics.com

I would like to thank all the authors for their willingness to contribute to this issue of *Clinics in Liver Disease*, Kerry Holland for her usual excellent editorial support in keeping authors (and the guest editor!) on schedule, and Dr. Norman Gitlin for giving me the opportunity to develop this edition.

Paul Martin, MD
Division of Hepatology
Schiff Liver Institute/Center for Liver Diseases
University of Miami
Miller School of Medicine
1500 NW 12 Avenue, Miami, FL 33136

E-mail address:
PMartin2@med.miami.edu (P. Martin)

The Asymptomatic Outpatient with Abnormal Liver Function Tests

Michael Krier, MD, Aijaz Ahmed, MD*

KEYWORDS

- Aminotransferases (ALT and AST) • LFT
- Alkaline phosphatase • Albumin • Prothrombin time

Traditionally, the constellation of biochemistry tests including liver enzymes, total bilirubin, and hepatic synthetic measures (prothrombin time (PT) and serum albumin level) are referred to as liver function tests (LFTs). Abnormal LFTs can be encountered during primary health care visits, routine blood donation, and insurance screening. A reported 1% to 4% of asymptomatic patients exhibit abnormal LFTs, leading to a sizeable number of annual consultations to a gastroenterology and/or hepatology practice.[1] A cost-effective and systematic approach is essential to the interpretation of abnormal LFTs.[2–7] A review of pattern of abnormal LFTs, detailed medical history, and a comprehensive physical examination help establish a foundation for further individualized testing. Further investigation often involves biochemical testing for disease-specific markers, radiographic imaging, and even consideration of a liver biopsy. In the following account, markers of hepatic injury are reviewed followed by a discussion on an approach to various patterns of abnormal LFTs in an asymptomatic patient.

ABNORMAL LFTS: MARKERS OF HEPATIC INJURY

Abnormal LFTs can be found in 2 main predominant patterns of hepatic injury, hepatocellular necrosis or cholestasis. Differentiation between these 2 main patterns of hepatic injury provides clues for further testing. However, in practice, patients present with a mixed pattern of hepatic injury.

Markers of Hepatocellular Injury

Aminotransferases

Alanine aminotransferase (ALT) and aspartate aminotransferase (AST) are normally intracellular enzymes with mitochondrial and cytoplasmic forms.[8] Their names reflect

Division of Gastroenterology and Hepatology, Stanford University School of Medicine, 750 Welch Road, Suite # 210, Stanford, CA 94304, USA
* Corresponding author.
E-mail address: aijazahmed@stanford.edu (A. Ahmed).

Clin Liver Dis 13 (2009) 167–177
doi:10.1016/j.cld.2009.02.001
1089-3261/09/$ – see front matter. Published by Elsevier Inc.

liver.theclinics.com

their role in catalyzing chemical reactions in which amino groups of alanine and aspartic acid are transferred to the alpha-keto group of ketoglutaric acid, particularly during gluconeogenesis. ALT and AST are widely distributed in cells throughout the body and are found in liver, heart, skeletal muscle, kidney, brain, and pancreas. ALT is exclusively cytoplasmic and is found primarily in the liver and kidney, with only minute amounts in heart and skeletal muscle.[8]

In addition to hepatic injury, there are many other factors that may affect aminotransferase serum levels. Hyperthyroidism has been noted to raise both AST and ALT levels. It has been postulated that excessive thyroid activity creates hepatic ischemia by increasing hepatic and splanchnic oxygen requirements.[9] Alcohol, in addition to being hepatotoxic, also stimulates mitochondrial AST activity, resulting in the release of mitochondrial AST from cells without measurable parenchymal damage.[8] Strenuous exercise can also raise AST values by 3-fold, and ALT has been found to be 20% lower in those who exercise regularly.[8] Both AST and ALT levels are 40% to 50% higher in individuals with a high BMI.[8] Muscle injury is associated with a significantly higher serum AST level (in contrast to ALT) in conditions such as rhabdomyolysis, polymyositis, and muscular dystrophy.[10–12] ALT levels demonstrate daily variation, lowest at night and highest in the afternoon.[8,13]

AST and ALT levels Absolute levels of aminotransferases correlate poorly with the severity or extent of hepatocellular damage and do not provide reliable prognostic information. Conversely, patients with a "burnt out" cirrhotic liver may have misleadingly low AST and ALT levels. However, the magnitude of enzyme levels categorized into mild, moderate, or markedly elevated levels can help differentiate between different causes of liver disease. Although a consensus on how to define these broad categories does not exist, many authorities would define mild elevation in aminotransferase levels as up to a 5-fold increase. A mild increase in AST or ALT levels can reflect both acute and chronic liver disease. Because of the obesity epidemic, it is likely that the most common reason for mild abnormalities in aminotransferases in the United States is nonalcoholic fatty liver disease (NAFLD).[14,15] In addition, a mild transaminitis can also reflect medications, alcoholic liver disease, viral hepatitis, autoimmune liver disease, celiac disease, and various metabolic/genetic diseases (Wilson's disease, alpha-1-antitrypsin deficiency, hemochromatosis, etc.). The category of high/marked elevation in aminotransferases includes a greater than 15-fold increase in levels (usually greater than 1000 U/L). When levels reach this magnitude, the differential diagnosis is narrowed to a fairly short list of conditions including acute viral hepatitis (A–E and herpes simplex virus [HSV]), ingestions (toxins/medications), and ischemic or "shock" liver. Rarely, other diagnoses to consider with marked elevations in aminotransferase levels include an acute exacerbation of autoimmune hepatitis, Budd-Chiari syndrome, HELLP (Hemolytic anemia, Elevated Liver enzymes, and Low Platelet count) syndrome, and Wilson's disease.[1] Aminotransferases greater than 100-fold are commonly noted in toxic injections (ie, acetaminophen) and ischemic liver injury but are rare in acute viral hepatitis.[8] Acute biliary ductal obstruction can transiently raise AST and ALT levels to greater than 15-fold, followed typically by cholestatic changes.[16]

AST/ALT ratio AST/ALT ratio can also provide an important diagnostic clue. The AST/ALT ratio in subjects without evidence of underlying liver disease is approximately 0.8. An AST/ALT ratio of 2.0 or greater and an absolute ALT level less than 300 U/L is suspicious of alcoholic liver disease. This distinctive pattern can be explained by 2 mechanisms. Patients with alcoholic liver disease often have a poor nutritional status leading to shortage of pyridoxal 5′-phosphate, which is a cofactor for both AST and ALT. Pyridoxal 5′-phosphate has a greater affinity for AST than ALT, resulting in significantly depressed ALT activity relative to AST. Second, alcohol induces plasma mitochondrial AST activity and stimulates release of mitochondrial AST, leading to further increase in the AST/ALT ratio.[8] However, patients with a history of significant alcohol use but no evidence of severe liver disease (alcoholic hepatitis or cirrhosis) will generally maintain an AST/ALT ratio less than 1.0.[17] In patients with other etiologies of liver disease, such as viral hepatitis, an AST/ALT ratio greater than 1.0 can be indicative of underlying cirrhosis with a high specificity (94%–100%), but a low sensitivity (44%–75%).[18] Patients with Wilson's disease can also manifest an AST/ALT ratio of greater than 4.0.[19,20] In contrast the AST/ALT ratio is usually 1.0 or less in NAFLD.[21]

Lactate dehydrogenase

Lactate dehydrogenase (LDH) has also been used to screen for liver disease. LDH is segmented into 5 isoenzyme forms (LDH-1 to LDH-5), with the latter of hepatic origin. The diagnostic sensitivity of LDH for liver disease is poor when compared with that of aminotransferases. Currently, LDH may be useful in specific instances, such as suggesting an ischemic hepatitis and in conjunction with a rising alkaline phosphatase (AP) level in infiltrative liver disease.

Markers of Cholestasis

Alkaline phosphatase

AP is found in many organs, including the placenta, ileal mucosa, kidney, bone, leukocytes, and liver.[22–29] AP is involved in phosphate ester hydrolysis, although its exact catalytic function is unknown. Liver and bone AP are the most abundant isoenzyme forms found in the serum and can be readily separated by electrophoretic measurements or heat treatment. Serum AP levels can rise as a result of either intrahepatic (primary biliary cirrhosis, primary sclerosing cholangitis, etc.) or extrahepatic (choledocholithiases, biliary stricture, etc.) biliary obstruction. This rise in serum AP level reflects de novo synthesis (induced by bile acid accumulation in hepatocytes rather than impairment of bile secretion).[28] As bile acids accumulate intracellularly, solubilization of the hepatic plasma membranes ensues, leading to AP release. Due to this mechanism (synthesis followed by release), a rise in serum AP level is often delayed by a few days following the onset of biliary obstruction. Serum AP has a half-life of 5 to 7 days and will remain elevated for several days despite resolution of biliary ductal obstruction. In addition to obstructive processes, infiltrative granulomatous or malignant (primary or metastatic) disease can result in a rise in AP levels due to compression and/or infiltration of small intrahepatic bile ducts. A tumor causing focal, infiltrative (intrahepatic), ductal obstruction may cause an isolated increase in AP levels without a concurrent rise in bilirubin. The converse can also be true with serum AP levels remaining normal in the setting of widespread metastatic disease or large-duct extrahepatic biliary obstruction.[29] In addition to hepatobiliary disease, several additional factors can affect AP serum levels. High-fat food intake can increase AP levels by 30 U/L; rise in BMI can increase AP levels by 25%; tobacco use can lead to 10% rise in AP levels; during the third trimester of pregnancy, AP levels can increase by 2- to 3-fold; and oral contraceptives can increase AP levels by 20%.[22–27] Chronic kidney disease has also been reported to raise serum levels of the intestinal AP isoenzyme.[24,25]

Gamma glutamyl transpeptidase

Hepatic gamma glutamyl transpeptidase (GGTP) is a microsomal enzyme found on the surface of hepatocytes and biliary epithelia. As with many microsomal enzymes,

GGTP is inducible. GGTP can be induced by alcohol, phenytoin, barbiturates, and warfarin. Clinically, its main utility is suggesting a hepatic source for an elevated AP.[18] However, it has a low predictive value (32%) for hepatobiliary disease, as it is present in numerous body compartments, including proximal renal tubule, pancreas (ductules and acinar cells), heart, lung, and brain.[8] Other clinical conditions in which GGTP elevation has been reported include diabetes mellitus, hyperthyroidism, rheumatoid arthritis, and chronic obstructive pulmonary disease.[30] In individuals with alcohol use, a GGTP/AP ratio of greater than 2.5 has been observed. However, its clinical utility in assessing surreptitious alcohol use is questionable, as it has a half-life of 26 days and demonstrates poor correlation with alcohol binging.[31] In addition, normal GGTP levels have been reported in more than one-third of subjects who consume more than 80 g of alcohol per day.

Bilirubin

Bilirubin is a catabolic end product from the breakdown of heme. The normal level is less than 1 mg/dL (18 μmol/L).[1] Elevated serum bilirubin levels generally reflect an imbalance between production and conjugation followed by excretion. Total bilirubin can be segmented further into a water-soluble form referred to as "direct/conjugated bilirubin" or a lipid-soluble form, namely, "indirect/unconjugated bilirubin." An elevation in direct bilirubin is highly specific for biliary tract obstruction. However, impaired biliary excretion, which is an energy-dependent process, is thought to be the reason for increased levels observed in sepsis, total parenteral nutrition, and following surgery.[32] Due to its small molecular size and water-soluble properties, direct bilirubin appears in urine.

Unconjugated Hyperbilirubinemia

A rise in unconjugated serum bilirubin levels reflects 2 basic pathophysiologic mechanisms, namely, bilirubin overproduction and reduced ability to conjugate bilirubin. Overproduction of unconjugated bilirubin occurs in hemolysis, ineffective erythropoiesis, large hematoma resorption, and extensive muscle injury. A personal or family history of anemia, recent blood transfusion, and a review of the patient's prescription medications may provide important diagnostic clues. A specific inquiry regarding the use of herbs, supplements, and other over-the counter nutritional or medicinal agents is important. Most cases of hemolysis cause only a modest rise (<5 mg/dL) in serum unconjugated bilirubin levels. However, severe hemolytic crises, including sickle cell disease and paroxysmal nocturnal hemoglobinuria, can markedly raise serum unconjugated bilirubin levels to greater than 30 mg/dL. At a minimum, an initial diagnostic evaluation for hemolysis should include a complete blood count, reticulocyte count, and an examination of peripheral blood smear. Second-tier tests to confirm hemolysis include LDH, haptoglobin, direct Coombs test, glucose-6-phosphate dehydrogenase assay, and hemoglobin electrophoresis. A rise in the level of unconjugated bilirubin can occur under any condition impairing effective blood return (and thus proper uptake and processing) back to the liver, such as congestive heart failure or portosystemic shunting (congenital or acquired). Finally, congenital conditions with defects in bilirubin conjugation, that is, Gilbert's or Crigler-Najjar syndrome, can cause increased unconjugated serum bilirubin levels.

Conjugated Hyperbilirubinemia

Conjugated hyperbilirubinemia is a total bilirubin with a direct bilirubin fraction greater than 50%. Etiologies causing conjugated hyperbilirubinemia are numerous but can be categorized under hepatocellular injury/necrosis and extrahepatic or intrahepatic cholestasis. The rate-limiting step in all these conditions is the inability of hepatocyte mass to excrete conjugated bilirubin either due to acquired or inherited defects. This process leads to accumulation of conjugated bilirubin and eventual "overflow" leakage into the serum.[33] The total bilirubin level provides prognostic information in patients with alcoholic hepatitis, primary biliary cirrhosis, and acute liver failure as well as in chronic liver disease and is one of the components of the Model for End-stage Liver Disease (MELD).[34,35]

Markers of Hepatic Synthetic Function

Prothrombin time

PT reflects the extrinsic clotting pathway involving factors II, V, VII, and X and is used to assess hepatic synthetic function. Factor VIII is the only clotting factor not synthesized by the liver but by vascular endothelium and reticuloendothelial cells. In addition to hepatic dysfunction of biliary obstruction, other explanations for a prolonged PT time include vitamin K deficiency, anticoagulation therapy, and consumption coagulopathy. In chronic liver disease, PT is generally within normal limits until progression to cirrhosis. In acute liver disease, PT is usually prolonged by at least 3 seconds in acute ischemic and toxic hepatitis, but, generally, it is not increased by more than 3 seconds in viral or alcoholic hepatitis.[36–39] A PT value greater than 100 seconds is part of King's College criteria for urgent liver transplantation in acute liver failure.[40] Monitoring of factor VII (half-life of 6 hours) can be useful to assess hepatic synthetic dysfunction in acute liver failure.[40] An International Normalized Ratio, a standardized measure of the patient PT to a control value, has been shown not to confer any additional prognostic advantage in the setting of acute liver failure.[41,42]

Albumin

Up to 10 g of albumin is normally produced and secreted each day by the liver. In advanced liver disease, PT and serum albumin level can be used to assess hepatic synthetic function. However, the half-life of plasma albumin is 20 days, which significantly reduces its utility for real-time assessment of hepatic synthetic function in acute liver disease. In addition, a number of other conditions may result in decreased serum albumin levels. These include excessive loss (protein-losing enteropathy, nephrotic syndrome, burn injury), increased turnover (hormonal dysfunction, glucocorticoids), and decreased intake (malnutrition). Prealbumin is also produced by the liver with a much shorter half-life (3 days) but is unfortunately affected by several other extrahepatic factors limiting its diagnostic utility.

ABNORMAL LFTS: ANALYSIS STRATEGY
History and Physical Examination

The approach to the asymptomatic patient with abnormal LFTs should always start with a detailed history and physical examination helping to quickly parse down a large number of etiologies. During a detailed history, important diagnostic clues can be obtained, including a complete medications list (new and old medications), herbs/homeopathic treatments (ma huang, chaparral, lady's mantle, shark cartilage, Scutellaria/skullcap, etc.), dietary agents (mushrooms, toxic ingestions, etc.), duration and amount of alcohol use, risk factors for viral hepatitis (history of blood transfusions, tattoos, intravenous drug use, etc.), sexual history, travel history, and family history. Information regarding country of origin can suggest a particular liver disease; for example, chronic hepatitis B is more prevalent in the Far East, schistosomiasis in Egypt, and malaria in Africa. During the physical examination, particular attention should be paid to stigmata of advance liver disease including firm liver edge, splenomegaly, ascites, asterixis, spider angiomata, palmar erythema, muscle wasting, and easy bruisability.

Approach to Asymptomatic Aminotransferase Elevation

An elevation in aminotransferase levels is a sensitive indicator of active hepatocellular inflammation and necrosis. A systematic approach to abnormal AST and ALT analysis should address the following key items: the rate of rise in enzyme elevation, the magnitude (enzyme peak) of rise, the AST/ALT ratio, and any other associated clinical stigmata of liver disease. Before ordering a battery of tests, any LFT abnormality should ideally be reconfirmed after a 2- to 3-month interval. However, higher initial LFT values correspond to a lower probability for false-positive values.[43] In patients with persistently elevated LFTs, a first-line approach to analysis should focus on attempts to uncover any reversible or potentially treatable causes (**Fig. 1**). In the United States, NAFLD is the most frequent cause of a mild transaminitis (up to 250 U/L) in the asymptomatic patient[44,45] and is suggested by uncovering risk factors or features of the metabolic syndrome. NAFLD is also prevalent in up to 10% to 15% of nonobese individuals, highlighting inherent diagnostic challenges.[46,47] An initial ultrasound of the liver can reveal a hyperechoic (bright) liver but may be false negative. The most frequent causes for mild-moderate transaminitis (250 to 1000 U/L) include viral hepatitis and hepatotoxic drugs. Viral etiologies include both the hepatotropic viruses (hepatitis virus A to E) and herpes viruses (Epstein-Barr, cytomegalovirus, and HSV),

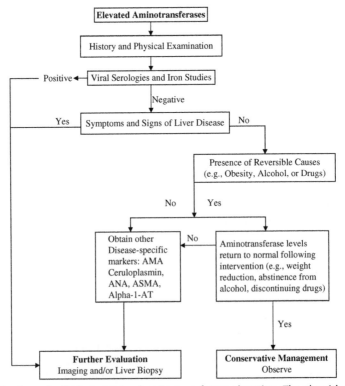

Fig. 1. Evaluation of mild but sustained aminotransferase elevation. The algorithm assumes elevation of both AST and ALT, making an extrahepatic source unlikely.

which can cause abnormal LFTs of this magnitude. The most common drug offenders include nonsteroidal anti-inflammatory agents, antiepileptics, antibiotics, statins, anabolic steroids, and recreational drugs of abuse, for example, cocaine, phencyclidine, glues, and solvents.

Hepatotoxic medications should be substituted or discontinued. An empiric trial of abstinence from alcohol should be initiated, and it can take up to several weeks to months for aminotransferases to return to normal. In patients with suspected NAFLD, sustained weight reduction should be encouraged to retard and possibly reverse fibrotic change. Further selective diagnostic testing includes serologic testing for hepatitis B and C; iron studies; checking serum ceruloplasmin in patients younger than 40 years to rule out Wilson's disease; checking serum protein electrophoresis in young females to rule out autoimmune hepatitis; obtaining thyroid-stimulating hormone levels; assessing creatine kinase levels; checking antibodies for celiac sprue; checking alpha-1-antitrypsin phenotype and levels; and searching for adrenocortical insufficiency (Addison's disease).[48,49]

Finally, if all the above diagnostic measures have been exhausted and LFTs remain persistently abnormal for 6 to 12 months, the following approach is suggested. First, if aminotransferase values are less than 1.5 times the upper limit of normal, observation may be reasonable. Secondly, with higher elevations in LFTs, a liver biopsy can provide valuable diagnostic and prognostic information.

Approach to Isolated or Predominant Alkaline Phosphatase Elevation

Predominance of liver AP elevation in the asymptomatic patient can most often be explained by either chronic cholestasis (partial biliary obstruction, primary biliary cirrhosis, primary sclerosing cholangitis, or drug-related cholestasis) or subtle infiltrative disease (granulomatous and malignancy). An initial step to evaluating abnormal AP levels should involve repeating the test under fasting conditions (**Fig. 2**). This step should be followed by organ identification, considering the lack of specificity of AP for the liver. Gel electrophoresis (isoenzyme determination) and heat separation methods are available for this purpose. However, simple measurement of a GGTP or 5'-nucleotidase is quicker and less expensive. These enzymes (GGTP or 5'-nucleotidase) parallel a rise in liver AP due to their disproportionately high concentration within liver and biliary epithelium. All suspected hepatotoxic medications should be discontinued. An ultrasound, antimitochondrial antibody, and other autoimmune markers should next be ordered to exclude extrahepatic ductal system (rare to be abnormally dilated without concomitant rise in bilirubin)/gross liver parenchymal abnormalities, primary biliary cirrhosis, overlap syndrome, or primary or secondary deposits in the liver. If no abnormalities are revealed and serum AP levels remain below 1.5-fold of normal, observation can be appropriate for these patients.[43] Finally, if significant AP elevation persists or if there is any further concern for the biliary structural (extra or intrahepatic) disease, a magnetic resonance cholangiopancreatography followed by an endoscopic retrograde cholangiopancreatography should be performed.

Isolated or Predominant GGTP Elevation

GGTP activity is inducible and can be elevated due to alcohol use, anticonvulsant medications, and warfarin. Age, gender, BMI, and smoking status can also influence GGTP levels.[50] However, an isolated GGTP distinctly raises the possibility of alcoholic liver disease. Alcohol avoidance for 2 to 3 months and follow-up GGTP testing is a reasonable approach in the absence of other evidence of liver disease.

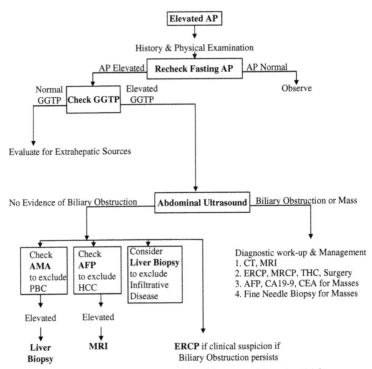

Fig. 2. Evaluation of isolated AP elevation. Clinical history taking should focus on excluding extrahepatic sources of AP (eg, symptoms of bone disease, pregnancy), medication use, symptoms of biliary colic, and cholestasis.

Drug-Induced Hepatotoxicity

Drug-induced hepatotoxicity is under-reported. It has an estimated incidence of 1:10,000 to 1:100,000.[51] However, in the United States, it is the leading cause (specifically acetaminophen) of acute liver failure[51,52] and drug withdrawal from the market.[53] Although many drugs are implicated in hepatotoxicity, common offenders include acetaminophen, methotrexate, and isoniazid. In addition, screening for hepatotoxicity has become a standard of care for certain medications, including statins, valproate, pyrazinamide, ketoconazole, dantrolene, tacrine, and synthetic retinoids. Clinical data on lipid-lowering agents, in particular statins, have provided assurance that mild transaminase elevations at baseline do not confer a higher risk for hepatotoxicity.[54]

Screening for drug-related hepatotoxicity is limited by a number of factors, including the lack of available commercial tests to accurately measure most drug levels, non–dose-related idiosyncratic reactions and risk of progressive hepatotoxicity despite persistently normal LFTs with the use of certain drugs, for example, long-term methotrexate. A liver biopsy can provide information regarding the severity and extent of histologic damage from drug-related injury.

ABNORMAL LFTS: SUMMARY

In summary, there is no ideal test or battery of studies to evaluate abnormal LFTs in an asymptomatic patient. Abnormal LFTs should be reconfirmed. Based on diagnostic clues obtained during clinical evaluation (detailed history, physical examination, a review of abnormally elevated LFTs, and other diagnostic data), an individualized diagnostic approach should be formulated. It may be crucial to plot a graph of duration, fluctuation, ratio, severity, and peak in LFT abnormalities and its relationship to exposure to potential hepatotoxic agents. A selective diagnostic approach appears cost effective and prudent in asymptomatic outpatients with abnormal LFTs.

REFERENCES

1. Green RM, Flamm S. AGA technical review on the evaluation of liver chemistry tests. Gastroenterology 2002;123:1367–84.
2. Prati D, Taioli E, Zanella A, et al. Updated definitions of healthy ranges for serum alanine aminotransferase levels. Ann Intern Med 2002;137:1–10.
3. Pratt DS, Kaplan MM. Laboratory tests. In: Schiff ER, Sorrell MF, Maddrey WC, editors, Schiff's diseases of the liver, vol. 1. Philadelphia: Lippincott-Raven; 1999. p. 205–44.
4. Kratz A, Lewandrowski KB. Case records of the Massachusetts General Hospital. Weekly clinicopathological exercises. Normal reference laboratory values. N Engl J Med 1998;339:1063–72.
5. Friedman LS, Martin P, Munoz SJ. Liver function tests and the objective evaluation of the patient with liver disease. In: Zakim D, Boyer TD, editors, Hepatology: a textbook of liver disease, vol. 1. Philadelphia: WB Saunders; 1996. p. 791–833.
6. Sackett DLHR, Guyatt GH, Tugwell P. Clinical epidemiology: a basic science for clinical medicine. Boston: Little Brown; 1991.
7. Henley KS, Schmidt FW, Schmidt E. Newer diagnostic tests in liver disease. In: Popper H, Schaffner F, editors. Progress in liver diseases, vol. 1. New York: Grune & Stratton; 1961. p. 216–28.
8. Dufour DR, Lott JA, Nolte FS, et al. Diagnosis and monitoring of hepatic injury. Recommendations for use of laboratory tests in screening, diagnosis, and monitoring of hepatic injury. Clin Chem 2000;46:2050–68.
9. Bayraktar M, Van Thiel DH. Abnormalities in measures of liver function and injury in thyroid disorders. Hepatogastroenterology 1997;44:1614–8.
10. Begum T, Oliver MR, Kornberg AJ, et al. Elevated aminotransferase as a presenting finding in a patient with occult muscle disease. J Paediatr Child Health 2000; 36:189–90.
11. Zamora S, Adams C, Butzner JD, et al. Elevated aminotransferase activity as an indication of muscular dystrophy: case reports and review of the literature. Can J Gastroenterol 1996;10:389–93.
12. Helfgott SM, Karlson E, Beckman E. Misinterpretation of serum transaminase elevation in "occult" myositis. Am J Med 1993;95:447–9.
13. Siest G, Schiele F, Galteau M-M, et al. Aspartate aminotransferase and alanine aminotransferase activities in plasma: statistical distributions, individual variations, and reference values. Clin Chem 1975;21:1077–87.
14. Reid AE. Nonalcoholic steatohepatitis. Gastroenterology 2001;121:710–23.
15. Bacon BR, Farahvash MJ, Janney CG, et al. Non-alcoholic steatohepatitis: an expanded clinical entity. Gastroenterology 1994;107:1103–9.
16. Fortson WC, Tedesco FJ, Starnes ED, et al. Marked elevation of serum transaminase activity associated with extrahepatic biliary tract disease. J Clin Gastroenterol 1985;7:502–5.
17. Nyblom H, Berggren U, Balldin J, et al. High AST/ALT ratio may indicate advanced alcoholic liver disease rather than heavy drinking. Alcohol Alcohol 2004;39:336–9.

18. Sorbi D, Boynton J, Lindor KD. The ratio of aspartate aminotransferase to alanine aminotransferase: potential value in differentiating nonalcoholic steatohepatitis from alcoholic liver disease. Am J Gastroenterol 1999;94:1018–22.
19. Berman DHLR, Gavaler JS, Cadoff EM, et al. Clinical differentiation of fulminant Wilsonian hepatitis from other causes of hepatic failure. Gastroenterology 1991; 100:1129–34.
20. Sallie R, Katsiyiannakis L, Baldwin D, et al. Failure of simple biochemical indexes to reliably differentiate fulminant Wilson's disease from other causes of fulminant liver failure. Hepatology 1992;16:1206–11.
21. Giboney PT. Mildly elevated liver transaminase levels in the asymptomatic patient. Am Fam Physician 2005;71:1105–10.
22. Lazo M, Selvin E, Clark JM. Brief communication: clinical implications of short-term variability in liver function test results. Ann Intern Med 2008;148:348–52.
23. Manolio TA, Burke GL, Savage PJ, et al. Sex- and race-related differences in liver-associated serum chemistry tests in young adults in the CARDIA study. Clin Chem 1992;28:1853–9.
24. Bayer PM, Hotschek H, Knoth E. Intestinal alkaline phosphatase and the ABO blood group system: a new aspect. Clin Chim Acta 1980;108:81–7.
25. Gordon T. Factors associated with serum alkaline phosphatase level. Arch Pathol Lab Med 1993;117:187–90.
26. Yamada N, Kido K, Hayashi S, et al. Characteristics of blood biochemical constituents of pregnant women. Acta Obstet Gynaecol Jpn 1977;29:447–50.
27. Dufour DR. Effects of oral contraceptives on routine laboratory tests. Clin Chem 1998;44(Suppl 6):A137.
28. Seetharam S, Sussman NL, Komoda T, et al. The mechanism of elevated alkaline phosphatase activity after bile duct ligation in the rat. Hepatology 1986;6:374–80.
29. McGarrity TJ, Samuels T, Wilson FA. An analysis of imaging studies and liver function tests to detect hepatic neoplasia. Dig Dis Sci 1987;32:1113–37.
30. Hedworth-Whitty RB, Whitfield JB, Richardson RW. Serum gamma-glutamyltranspeptidase activity in myocardial ischaemia. Br Heart J 1967;29:432–8.
31. Penn R, Worthington DJ. Is serum gamma-glutamyltransferase a misleading test? Br Med J 1983;286:531–5.
32. Zimmerman HJ. Intrahepatic cholestasis. Arch Intern Med 1979;139:1038–45.
33. Scharschmidt BF, Blanckaert N, Farina FA, et al. Measurement of serum bilirubin and its mono- and diconjugates: application to patients with hepatobiliary disease. Gut 1982;23:643–9.
34. Kamath PS, Wiesner RH, Malinchoc M, et al. A model to predict survival in patients with end-stage liver disease. Hepatology 2001;33:464–70.
35. Wiesner R, Edwards E, Freeman R, et al. The United Network for Organ Sharing Liver Disease Severity Score Committee. Model for end-stage liver disease (MELD) and allocation of donor livers. Gastroenterology 2003;124:91–6.
36. Fuchs S, Bogomolski-Yahalom V, Paltiel O, et al. Ischemic hepatitis: clinical and laboratory observations of 34 patients. J Clin Gastroenterol 1998;26:183–6.
37. Singer AJ, Carracio TR, Mofenson HC. The temporal profile of increased transaminase levels in patients with acetaminophen-induced liver dysfunction. Ann Emerg Med 1995;26:49–53.
38. Willner IR, Uhl MD, Howard SC, et al. Serious hepatitis A: an analysis of patients hospitalized during an epidemic in the United States. Ann Intern Med 1998;128: 111–4.
39. Mendenhall CL, VA Cooperative Study Group on Alcoholic Hepatitis. Alcoholic hepatitis. Clin Gastroenterol 1981;10:417–41.

40. O'Grady JG, Alexander GJ, Hayllar KM, et al. Early indicators of prognosis in fulminant hepatic failure. Gastroenterology 1989;97:439–45.
41. Kovacs MJ, Wong A, MacKinnon K, et al. Assessment of the validity of the INR system for patients with liver impairment. Thromb Haemost 1994;71:727–30.
42. Denson KW, Reed SV, Haddon ME. Validity of the INR system for patients with liver impairment. Thromb Haemost 1995;73:162.
43. Pratt DS, Kaplan MM. Evaluation of abnormal liver-enzyme results in asymptomatic patients. N Engl J Med 2000;342:1266–71.
44. Clark JM, Brancati FL, Diehl AM. The prevalence and etiology of elevated aminotransferase levels in the United States. Am J Gastroenterol 2003;98:960–7.
45. Patt CH, Yoo HY, Dibadj K, et al. Prevalence of transaminase abnormalities in asymptomatic, healthy subjects participating in an executive health-screening program. Dig Dis Sci 2003;48:797–801.
46. Christoffersen P, Petersen P. Morphological features in noncirrhotic livers from patients with chronic alcoholism, diabetes mellitus or adipositas. A comparative study. Acta Pathol Microbiol Scand [A] 1978;86A:495–8.
47. Tominaga K, Kurata JH, Chen YK, et al. Prevalence of fatty liver in Japanese children and relationship to obesity. An epidemiological ultrasonographic survey. Dig Dis Sci 1995;40:2002–9.
48. Boulton R, Hamilton MI, Dhillon AP, et al. Subclinical Addison's disease: a cause of persistent abnormalities in transaminase values. Gastroenterology 1995;109:1324–7.
49. Bardella MT, Vecchi M, Conte D, et al. Chronic unexplained hypertransaminasemia may be caused by occult celiac disease. Hepatology 1999;29:654–7.
50. Conigrave KM, Degenhardt LJ, Whitfield JB, et al. CDT, GGT, and AST as markers of alcohol use: the WHO/ISBRA collaborative project. Alcohol Clin Exp Res 2002;26:332–9.
51. Navarro VJ, Senior JR. Drug-related hepatotoxicity. N Engl J Med 2006;354:731–9.
52. Ostapowicz G, Lee WM. Acute hepatic failure: a Western perspective. J Gastroenterol Hepatol 2000;15:480–8.
53. Andrade RJ, Lucena MI, Fernandez MC, et al. Drug-induced liver injury: an analysis of 461 incidences submitted to the Spanish registry over a 10-year period. Gastroenterology 2005;129:512–21.
54. Chalasani N, Aljadhey H, Kesterson J, et al. Patients with elevated liver enzymes are not at higher risk for statin hepatotoxicity. Gastroenterology 2004;126:1287–92.

The Hospitalized Patient with Abnormal Liver Function Tests

Christopher B. O'Brien, MD, FACG

KEYWORDS

- Hospitalized • Evaluation • Liver function tests • LFTs
- Operation risk calculation

An inpatient consultation often asks a specific question such as "What is the operative risk in this patient?" Or, on occasion, the inpatient consultation may be a more general request such as "Patient known to you, please evaluate."

The most useful impression on the consultation form regarding abnormal LFTs in a hospitalized patient should comment on the following: (1) *chronicity*: for example, acute decompensation of chronically abnormal liver function tests (LFTs); (2) *etiology* of the patient's liver disease: acute ischemic hepatopathy superimposed on chronic nonalcoholic steatohepatitis; (3) *severity* of the process: cirrhosis: Child's C; Model for End-Stage Liver Disease (MELD) score 22; 80% operative risk in abdominal surgery of mortality; and (4) *complications*: + ascites, + encephalopathy, + esophageal varices, needs screening for hepatocellular carcinoma.

OVERVIEW OF PROCESS

The evaluation of abnormal LFTs in a hospitalized patient tends to assume more urgency than that in the outpatient setting. The preliminary step is a determination as to whether the abnormal LFTs are associated with the initial reason for the patient's hospitalization, are secondary to a chronic underlying liver disease preceding the admission, or developed in hospital. A careful history, either directly from the patient or family members, a review of outpatient records, and/or phone calls to the patient's physician may be critical in providing the necessary information.

Evaluation of the underlying etiology of the liver disease is the second step. If the abnormal LFTs in question is an isolated aminotransferase elevation, then confirmation of the source of the serum enzyme, whether of hepatic origin or elsewhere, is important.

The third step is to determine the acuteness or severity of the dysfunction. The methods for calculating the severity depend on whether the inpatient admission is associated with de novo acute liver failure (ALF) or acute decompensation of *chronic* liver

---

Divisions of Liver and Gastrointestinal Transplantation, Center for Liver Diseases, University of Miami Miller School of Medicine, 1500 NW 12th Avenue, Suite #1101 Miami, FL 33136, USA
E-mail address: cobrien@med.miami.edu

Clin Liver Dis 13 (2009) 179–192
doi:10.1016/j.cld.2009.02.010
1089-3261/09/$ – see front matter © 2009 Elsevier Inc. All rights reserved.

disease. If acute, then the King's College Criteria for Liver Transplantation or the MELD score may be most appropriate. Conversely, in the case of a chronic presentation of underlying liver disease, the procedure should be assessing the stage (severity) of fibrosis. If stage 4 fibrosis (cirrhosis) is present, then a MELD score (**Fig. 1**) is calculated to determine whether the patient needs liver transplant evaluation during this admission.

The final and fourth step is to look for any associated complications resulting from the presence of either the acute or chronic liver disease.

STEP 1: HISTORY AND PHYSICAL EXAMINATION
History

A meticulous medical history focused on the liver can provide important clues regarding abnormal LFTs in the hospitalized patient. Of utmost importance, yet frequently over-looked, is the determination as to whether the patient had pre-existing abnormal LFTs before the recent illness and hospitalization. In particular, it must be determined whether the liver disease has occurred suddenly, developed gradually, or simply has not been apparent until the hospitalization.

Clues that can be helpful for suggesting specific causes include the presence of right upper quadrant pain, fever, and nausea $\pm$ vomiting, all of which are suggestive of possible biliary tract disease. A history of intravenous drug use and recent foreign travel, associated with a viral prodrome, would raise the likelihood of an acute viral hepatitis. A history of previous liver disease or surgeries involving the liver can also offer important information. Careful questioning about consumption of alcohol, frequency, and amount from both the patient as well as the family can also be helpful. However, by far, the most important comment of the history is accurate information on medication use (whether prescription, illicit, or herbal) and the time course in relation to the hepatic dysfunction.

Calculation of the model for end-stage liver disease (MELD) score

MELD Score =	0.957 x Loge(creatinine mg/dL)
	+ 0.378 x Loge(bilirubin mg/dL)
	+ 1.120 x Loge(INR)
	+ 0.643*

INR, international normalized ratio

The maximum serum creatinine level in the MELD score equation is 4.0 mg/dL

Multiply by 10 and round to the nearest whole number

Laboratory values less than 1.0 are set to 1.0 for the purposes of the MELD score

calculation.

Fig. 1. Calculation of the model for end-stage liver disease (MELD) score. The maximum serum creatinine level in the MELD score equation is 4.0 mg/dL. Multiply by 10 and round to the nearest whole number. Laboratory values less than 1.0 are set to 1.0 for the purposes of the MELD score calculation. INR, International normalized ratio.

Physical Examination

Often forgotten in this age of high technology is that a thorough physical examination can often shed light on the cause, severity, and, occasionally, presence of 1 or more complications of liver disease. It has been said that "One good feel of the liver is worth any 2 LFTs" (F.M. Hanger Jr., 1971). Above all, it should be noted whether the liver is large or small, soft/hard, or nodular and whether tenderness is present over the liver itself or in the region of the gallbladder. A tender liver would suggest acute enlargement secondary to congestion, hepatitis, or cholangitis.

In particular, signs of right-sided heart failure including jugular venous distention, an enlarged tender liver, tricuspid regurgitation murmur, clubbing, an increased pulmonary heart sound, or fixed splitting of the second heart sound (suggestive of pulmonary hypertension), could suggest either acute or chronic hepatic congestion and/or the presence of the hepatopulmonary syndrome. The presence or absence of abdominal scars, palpable abdominal masses, or lymphadenopathy can also be helpful.

Characteristic changes should be sought on physical examination for chronicity of the liver disease, such as jaundice, scleral icterus, muscle wasting, spider angiomata, palmar erythema, splenomegaly, prominent abdominal pains, ascites, pedal edema, and a hepatic encephalopathy (asterixis). Additional findings include gynecomastia, fetor hepaticus, xanthelasmas, Dupuytren's contractures, and caput medusa.

STEP 2: LABORATORY EVALUATION FOR ETIOLOGY
Blood Panels

Liver function tests

Confirming hepatic origin Of concern, especially in the case of an isolated enzyme elevation, is to ensure that the abnormal LFT in question is of hepatic origin. Common liver enzymes, such as aspartame aminotransferase (AST) are found not only in the liver but can also derive from cardiac muscle, skeletal muscle, kidneys, brain, pancreas, lungs, and erythrocytes.[1] Other causes of serum AST elevation are rhabdomyolysis, recent vigorous physical activity, or inflammatory muscle disease. In a similar fashion, an elevated alkaline phosphatase may not only indicate a hepatobiliary origin but can also frequently point to a bone or intestinal source (in particular in patients with blood type O or B after the ingestion of a fatty meal).[2] Therefore, the serum alkaline phosphatase level is best determined in the fasting state. A serum albumin level is usually used to indicate overall liver function; an abnormally low serum albumin level may reflect disease in another organ system, such as a protein-losing enteropathy or nephrotic syndrome.

The best approach to an isolated LFT abnormality such as alkaline phosphatase would be to order isoenzymes fractionation.[3] Macroenzymes are molecules of high molecular weight, which are formed by the binding of a normal enzyme to another plasma protein, and have most commonly been described with isolated AST elevations.[4]

Evaluation of the LFT pattern Evaluation of the pattern of the initial LFT panel (**Table 1**) in association with serum prothrombin time and platelet count is key.[5] Although characteristic changes are not always present, this can provide a useful initial guidance, which can be confirmed by disease-specific blood testing, radiographic imaging, or liver biopsy.

The first determination is whether the pattern is more characteristic of "hepatitis" or cholestasis.[6] The predominant "hepatitis" pattern with alanine aminotransferase (ALT) and AST elevation out of proportion to alkaline phosphatase is characteristic of viral

Table 1
Patterns of liver function tests according to cause of liver disease

	Hepatocellular			Biliary		Infiltration
	Ischemia, & Toxins	Viral Hepatitis	Alcohol	Complete	Partial	Infiltrative Disease
Aminotransferases	50–100×	5–50×	2–5×	1–5×	1–5×	1–3×
Alk phos	1–3×	1–3×	1–10×	2–20×	2–10×	1–20×
Bilirubin	1–5×	1–30×	1–30×	1–30×	1–5×	1–5×
Prothrombin time	Prolonged and unresponsive to vitamin K in severe disease			Responsive to SQ vitamin K		Usually nl
Albumin	Decreased chronic disease			Usually nl		Usually nl
Platelet count	Decrease suggests stage III/IV			Usually nl		Usually nl

Abbreviations: Alk phos, alkaline phosphatase; nl, normal; SC, subcutaneous.
Data from Aijaz A, Keeffe EB. Liver Chemistry and function tests. In: Feldman, Friedman, Brandt, editors. Sleisenger & Fordtran's gastrointestinal and liver disease. 8th edition. Philadelphia: Saunders Elsevier; 2006. p. 1575–86.

hepatitis, nonalcoholic steatohepatitis, and alcohol- and drug-induced liver disease. A serum ALT to AST ratio greater than 2:1, but where the AST is less than 10 times the upper limit of normal, is consistent with alcoholic liver disease.[7]

If the pattern is cholestatic, then it is important to differentiate extrahepatic biliary tract obstruction from intrahepatic cholestasis. Classical biliary of the alkaline phosphatase elevation includes biliary strictures, choledocholithiasis, primary sclerosing cholangitis, and cholangiocarcinoma. Causes of the intrahepatic cholestasis include drug-induced etiologies, granulomatous disease and primary biliary cirrhosis, and malignant infiltration of the liver.[6] An elevated alkaline phosphatase is not invariable with neoplastic liver disease.[8]

Platelet count and prothrombin time

Jaundice in the face of a high platelet count is suggestive of acute liver disease or metastatic cancer/lymphoma involving liver. An elevation in the AST much greater than that in ALT is suggestive of shock liver as is a rapid rise in the serum prothrombin time, returning to normal over a period of several days. Acute acetaminophen toxicity can present with a significant elevation in the prothrombin time out of proportion to the elevation in the total bilirubin. Subcutaneous vitamin K will normalize the prothrombin time in patients with extrahepatic biliary obstruction but usually not with intrahepatic cholestasis. Chronically low platelet count (in the absence of bone marrow suppression or increased consumption) raises the possibility of liver fibrosis (stage 3 or 4) with portal hypertension and secondary hypersplenism.

Serologic testing

Following the evaluation of the LFTs, other blood tests are ordered to test for various etiologies of liver disease (**Box 1**). Depending on whether the liver test abnormalities were present before admission to the hospital, testing should also be sent for blood toxicology screens (especially on admission to the emergency room), viral liver disease, autoimmune hepatitis, primary sclerosing cholangitis, hemochromatosis, nonalcoholic fatty liver disease (NAFLD), and, if indicated by age, Wilson's disease (**Table 2**).

Box 1
Initial laboratory testing

Recommended Initial Testing

Toxicology testing (in emergency room/ day 1 of hospitalization)

    Urine and blood toxicology screens

Viral

    Hepatitis A antibody (IgM)

    Hepatitis B surface antigen, hepatitis B core antibody total, and surface antibody

    Hepatitis C antibody

Viral (optional)

    If hepatitis B surface antigen (+)

        Hepatitis viral B DNA (PCR)

        Hepatitis B antigen and antibody

    If hepatitis C antibody (+)

        Hepatitis viral C RNA (PCR) and genotype

    If immunosuppressed (future: microarray panel testing)

        Cytomegalovirus antibody (IgM)

        Epstein-Barr viral antibody (IgM)

        Herpes simplex antibody (IgM)

Auto antibodies

    Antinuclear antibody

    Antismooth muscle antibody

    Antimitochondrial antibody

    Perinuclear anti-neutrophil cytoplasmic antibody (atypical)

Metabolic

    Ceruloplasmin (serum), urine for 24-h copper

    Ferritin, iron, total iron-binding capacity

    Fasting insulin, lipid profile, hemoglobin A_{1c}

Abbreviations: IgM, immunoglobulin M; PCR, polymerase chain reaction.

Noninvasive Evaluation Techniques

Noninvasive radiographic imaging is the next procedure to supplement the results of blood testing.

Radiographic imaging

Ultrasound/Doppler ultrasound Abdominal ultrasound (US), with or without a Doppler ultrasound (DUS) component, is usually the initial imaging test in the evaluation of hepatobiliary disease. Important information gleaned from the US report may be the presence of hepatic masses as well as information about the diameter of the extrahepatic biliary tree. A caveat, however, is that patients with significant cirrhosis of the liver, especially due to primary sclerosing cholangitis or primary biliary cirrhosis, may have less biliary tract dilatation than would normally be expected with acute biliary

Table 2
Etiologies of acute and chronic liver disease

Liver Disease Classification	
Viral (classical)	Metabolic
Hepatitis A	Wilson's disease
Hepatitis B	Hemochromatosis
Hepatitis C	Steatosis (NASH/NAFL)
Hepatitis D	Pregnancy
Hepatitis E	
Viral (other)	Alcohol
Cytomegalovirus	Autoimmune hepatitis
Epstein-Barr virus	Ischemic
Herpes simplex virus	Arterial thrombosis
	Budd-Chiari syndrome
	Veno-occlusive disease
Medications	Malignancy
Prescription	Primary
Illicit	Hepatocellular carcinoma
Herbal	Cholangiocarcinoma
	Metastatic
Biliary	Unknown etiology
Choledocholithiasis	Primary sclerosing cholangitis
Biliary stricture	Primary biliary cirrhosis
Choledochocele(s)	
AIDS cholangiopathy	

Abbreviation: NASH, nonalcoholic steatohepatitis.

tract obstruction.[9] With these exceptions, nevertheless, the overall sensitivity of US for the detection of biliary obstruction in the presence of jaundice is around 90% with comparable specificity.[10]

Computed tomography and magnetic resonance imaging Computed Tomography (CT) is clearly superior to US for detection of intrahepatic and extrahepatic masses, as well as providing superior information about other organs of the abdominal region. However, in a patient with a high suspicion of biliary tract disease, magnetic resonance cholangiopancreatography (MRCP) is clearly superior to CT in the evaluation of the biliary system and determining the cause of possible obstruction.

The contour of the liver, in particular the presence of modularity as well as caudate lobe enlargement, correlates with the presence of cirrhosis on liver biopsy.[11] The presence of splenomegaly, dilatation of the portal vein, paraesophageal, and/or gastric varices can also be useful to suggest the presence of portal hypertension.

Nuclear medicine
DISIDA Scan Previously, hepatobiliary scintigraphy initially with hepatobiliary iminodiacetic acid (HIDA) scan, now more commonly the diisopropyl iminodiacetic acid (DISIDA) scan, was used to seek for biliary tract obstruction. However, given the superior information available with modern CT and MRI/MRCP imaging techniques, it is no longer recommended as an initial examination. In addition, accurate information from a DISIDA scan is limited to patients with a serum bilirubin level less than 20 mg/dL. The DISIDA scan remains sensitive, however, for the evaluation of the presence of acute cholecystitis or for a potential bile leak after biliary tract surgery or an endoscopic retrograde cholangiopancreatography (ERCP) sphincterotomy.[12]

Liver spleen scans Ninety percent of sulfur colloid tagged with technetium-99 m is removed by the liver, with the remaining particles extracted by the spleen and bone marrow. The ratio of the sulfur colloid clearance by the spleen and bone marrow increases in proportion to that by the liver with worsening liver function.[13] In addition, abnormal (patchy) distribution of the sulfur colloid is found in patients with severe liver disease. Despite improvements in the technique with Technetium-99 m, single-positron emission computed tomography (SPECT) scanning computer reconstruction of the image, this has fallen out of favor with better imaging of liver by CT and MRI scans.[14]

Endoscopic Techniques

Endoscopic ultrasound
Endoscopic ultrasound (EUS) is a newer technique with increasing use over the last several years. Overall, it has a sensitivity and specificity similar to those of MRCP.[15] However, it also has the advantage of permitting biopsy of suspected areas of malignancy.[16]

Endoscopic retrograde cholangiopancreatography
ERCP is the classic endoscopic method for the evaluation of the biliary system and the associated pancreatic duct. Among its advantages is its high degree of accuracy, with sensitivity rates of 89% to 90% and specificity rates of 89% to 100%.[10] The disadvantage is that it is an invasive procedure with a risk of complications both related to performance of endoscopy as well as specific to the injection and manipulation of the biliary tree and pancreatic duct.[17] A study comparing available techniques found sensitivity and specificity for diagnosis of malignancy in patients: 85% to 75% for ERCP, 85% to 71% for MRCP, 77% to 63% for CT, and 79% to 62% for EUS.[15]

Specific Patterns and Considerations

Acute biliary tract disease
Choledocholithiasis and biliary stricture Acute bile duct obstruction produces an elevation of alkaline phosphatase out of proportion to the serum aminotransferases. However, early in acute biliary obstruction, the AST and ALT may transiently rise as high as 10 to 20 times the upper limit of normal.[18] US is sensitive in the presence of biliary dilatation; however, it is much less sensitive in the presence of a nondilated bile duct. Confirmatory investigations include EUS, MRCP, and ERCP. A National Institutes of Health consensus statement concluded that the EUS, MRCP, and ERCP have comparable sensitivity and specificity in the detection of common bile duct stones.[19]

Specific hepatocellular diseases and patterns
Infectious hepatitis ALF in the United States is most commonly due to drug hepatotoxicity. However, acute viral liver disease including hepatitis A, hepatitis B and, extremely rarely, superinfection with hepatitis D or acute hepatitis E must also be considered.[20]

In patients on immunosuppression, particularly post-transplant, the herpes viruses (Epstein-Barr virus, cytomegalovirus, varicella zoster virus, and the herpes simplex virus) must also be kept in mind. Newer simultaneous DNA microarray technology may make a rapid diagnosis in the future in this setting.[21]

In addition to viral etiologies, abnormal LFTs commonly occur in the inpatient in the presence of disseminated infection, in particular both gram-negative and gram-positive bacterial infection. However, abnormal LFTs with other infections, including spirochetal, protozoal, fungal, and helminthic, can also occur.

Associated with malignancy Primary hepatobiliary carcinoma as well as liver infiltration by metastatic disease frequently causes abnormal LFTs. Metastases are more common than primary malignant tumors of the liver. Standard LFTs do not discriminate between primary and metastatic carcinomas. The various imaging modalities discussed earlier are the best means to further evaluate suspected malignant involvement of the liver.

Drug-induced liver injury Although many drugs in the Physician Desk Reference have been associated with abnormal LFTs, certain classes of medication are more frequently linked than others. In addition to prescription medications, herbal medications, illegal recreational substances, and environmental toxins have also been associated with drug-induced liver injury (DILI). The most common class of drug hepatotoxicity encountered during hospitalization is reaction to a medication, especially anti-microbial drugs.[22] However, multiple other classes of drugs have also been implicated. (For further information, please see Chapter 7: Modern Hepatotoxicity) DILI can, in general, be grouped into 1 of 2 presentations: predictable and idiosyncratic hepatotoxicity. Hepatotoxins frequently have a characteristic pattern of liver test abnormality: hepatitis, cholestatic, or mixed.

Predictable hepatotoxicity

In predictable hepatotoxicity, the presentation is directly related to the dose of the drug received and tends to develop almost immediately with necrosis in zone 3 of the liver.[23] This is not due to the drug itself but most commonly secondary to a metabolite. An example of this would be acetaminophen.[24] The Acute Liver Failure Study Group suggests that the majority of cases (39%) of ALF, one of the most dreaded complications of liver disease, are due to acetaminophen overdose.[24] In the acetaminophen group, there was a 68% chance of spontaneous survival, with only 6% of patients undergoing liver transplantation.

Idiosyncratic (unpredictable) hepatotoxicity

In contrast, the onset of liver dysfunction associated with an idiosyncratic drug reaction tends to be slower.[25] This reaction occurs rarely, is more common after multiple exposures, and is unrelated to the dose of the drug. Occasionally, it can be associated with fever, rash, and eosinophilia. However, ALF due to idiosyncratic drug reactions clearly has had a more dismal prognosis, with an overall 25% survival and up to 53% of patients requiring liver transplantation.[24]

The best way to determine whether a medication is responsible for the abnormal LFT is to stop that particular medication and determine if the LFTs return to normal.[26] Occasionally, this is not possible in an acute, rapidly deteriorating situation, in which case, a liver biopsy may be necessary to help identify which drug is most likely responsible.

Ischemic hepatitis Ischemic hepatitis is a common cause within the hospital of extreme AST elevation greater than 2000 U/L.[27] One of the most common etiologies is cardiovascular disease, which is reported to be responsible for almost 70% of cases.[28] Acute liver ischemia can result from generalized hypotension, particularly in the presence of underlying cirrhosis of the liver. It is not uncommon for the prothrombin time to be acutely prolonged over a rapid return to normal within the space of 2 to 3 days, followed by the serum aminotransferase levels within 7 to 10 days.

In addition, however, hypoxia, hyperthermia, and acute vascular occlusive disease can also present with acute abnormalities in LFTs, resulting in the need for hospitalization. In addition, acute hepatic vein thrombosis (Budd-Chiari syndrome) can result in sudden onset of ascites and hepatic decompensation.

Alcoholic liver disease Many patients conceal alcohol abuse, and, therefore, the diagnosis of alcoholic liver disease is not always obvious. Patients present with an AST to ALT ratio of at least 2:1.[29] This should slowly improve during a prolonged hospitalization. In addition, although not commonly used within the hospital after the first few days of admission, is the carbohydrate-deficient transferrin. Although it is a relative specific marker for alcohol abuse, it tends to decline after the patient has been absent for 4 days.[30] (For further information, please see Chapter 8: Management of Alcoholic Liver Disease.)

Jaundice in the postoperative period Postoperative jaundice is often multifactorial. However, abnormal LFTs can occur in almost 25% to 75% of patients postsurgery.[31] Although this can happen in patients with completely normal liver function preoperatively, this tends to be more common in patients with compensated cirrhosis (almost 50% of the patients).[32] A number of additional factors include impaired liver perfusion due to intraoperative or postoperative hypotension/hypoxia, blood transfusions, medication reactions, and occult sepsis. (For further information, see Chapter 4: Surgery in the Patient with Liver Disease).

Chronic liver disease Finally, all forms of chronic liver disease can, of course, be diagnosed for the first time during admission to the hospital. In fact, the most common etiology of liver disease in the United States at the present time is NAFLD.[33]

STEP 3: EVALUATION OF SEVERITY
Acute Liver Disease (Prognostic Factors)

King's College Criteria
The King's College Criteria were initially reported to be effective in providing prognostic of the need for liver transplantation in ALF due to acetaminophen (**Table 3**).[34] The criteria, however, were later modified to include ALF secondary to other etiologies. Moreover, in nonacetaminophen-related ALF, the presence of even a single adverse prognostic factor (see **Table 3**) predicts mortality of 80%.[35]

Chronic Liver Disease Liver With/Without Acute Decompensation
Since chemistry panels are commonly ordered as part of the initial admission to the hospital, many chronic liver diseases can be recognized for the first time. The causes of chronic liver disease are listed in **Table 2**.

Table 3	
King's College Criteria for transplantation in acute liver failure	
Nonacetaminophen Cases	**Acetaminophen Cases**

INR >6.5 (PT >100 s) or any 3 of the following:
  Idiosyncratic drug/indeterminant
  Age <10 or >40 y
  Acute/subacute presentation
  Serum bilirubin >17.5 mg/dL
  INR >3.5 (PT >50 s)
	Arterial pH <7.3 or any 1 of the following:
	  Stage III/IV encephalopathy
	  Serum creatinine >3.4 mg/dL
	  INR >6.5 (PT >100 s)

Abbreviations: INR, international normalized ratio; PT, prothrombin time.
   Data from O'Grady JG, Alexander GJ, Hayllar KM, et al. Early indicators of prognosis in fulminant hepatic failure. Gastroenterology 1989;97:439-45; and Bernal W, Donaldson N, Wyncoll D, et al. Blood lactate as an early predictor of outcome in paracetamol-induced acute liver failure: a cohort study. Lancet 2002;359:558–63.

Child-Turcotte-Pugh

The Child-Turcotte-Pugh (CTP) classification was initially used to predict mortality postcholecystectomy (**Table 4**). Its use has been generalized to the prognosis of patients postabdominal surgery (**Table 5**) of all types.[36] Surgery is always contraindicated in patients with Child's class C cirrhosis unless a life-threatening indication is present, such as bowel infarction, gangrenous cholecystitis, or incarcerated hernia. The estimation of operative risk in patients with cirrhosis was previously based on the Child-Turcotte-Pugh score, which has now been replaced by the Model for End-Stage Liver Disease (MELD).

MELD Score

The MELD scoring system was initially developed to predict 3-month mortality in patients undergoing transjugular intrahepatic portosystemic shunts.[37] The MELD scoring system is based on the serum bilirubin level, international normalized ratio (INR), and the serum creatinine level (see **Fig. 1**). This was adopted in February 2002 as the primary determinant for organ allocation in the United States. MELD is useful in predicting 3-month mortality in patients before and after transplant.[38]

Evaluation of Operative Risk

Elective surgical procedures are contraindicated in the face of active liver disease until a complete evaluation has been undertaken. In general, patients can be classified into those with minimal operative risk and those with increased operative risk, which includes those of active hepatitis and cirrhosis.

Child-Turcotte-Pugh

The CTP classification was initially used to predict mortality postcholecystectomy (see **Table 4**). Its use has been generalized for prognosis of all cirrhotic patients (see **Table 5**).[36]

Model for end-stage liver disease

The MELD scoring system has also been also applied to predict the outcome after surgery in cirrhotic patients.[39] It has the advantage of being more objective than the CTP classification, which is limited by subjective grading of some variables, such as ascites and hepatic encephalopathy. In addition, the CTP is unable to provide adequate risk assessment in patients with severely decompensated liver disease. (For further information, see the article by O'Leary and colleagues elsewhere in this issue.)

Table 4
Calculation of the Child-Turcotte-Pugh classification

Parameter	Numerical Score		
	1	2	3
Ascites	None	Slight	Moderate/severe
Encephalopathy	None	Slight/moderate	Moderate/severe
Bilirubin (mg/dL)	<2.0	2.1–3	≥3.1
Albumin (g/dL)	≥3.5	2.8–3.5	≤2.7
Prothrombin time (s)[a]	1–4	4.1–6	>6.0

Grade (A): 5–6, grade (B): 7–9, grade (C): 10–15.
[a] seconds increased over control.

Table 5 Child-Turcotte-Pugh score and predicted operative mortality		
Total Numerical Score	**Child-Turcotte-Pugh Class**	**Operative Mortality Rate**
5–6	A	10%
7–9	B	30%
10–15	C	82%

The Mayo Clinic has made a recent modification to the MELD score that calculates the postoperative day 7, day 30, day 90, year 1, and year 5 in patients with cirrhosis for all types of major surgery. This model includes in addition to bilirubin level, creatinine level, and INR, the American Society of Anesthesiologists classification and the etiology of disease (http://www.mayoclinic.org/meld/mayomodel9.html).

STEP 4: EVALUATION FOR COMPLICATIONS
Acute Liver Failure

This rare clinical syndrome is defined as development of coagulopathy in association with hepatic encephalopathy within 26 weeks of recognition of liver disease in a patient without pre-existing liver disease. Causes of death include sepsis, hypoglycemia, cerebral edema, multisystem organ failure, acute respiratory distress syndrome, and renal failure (acute tumor necrosis and type 1 hepatorenal syndrome). Bacterial infections develop in as many as 80% of patients.[40]

Chronic Liver Disease

Sometimes a complication of chronic liver disease can be one of the major reasons for the patient's admission to the hospital. Alternatively, a patient with chronic liver disease is admitted for another reason. During the hospital admission, the patient may be noted to have thrombocytopenia. If the subsequent evaluation suggests cirrhosis, it is helpful to look for the presence of a complication of cirrhosis. These typically include esophageal or gastric varices, ascites, hepatic encephalopathy, and hepatocellular carcinoma. However, it should not be forgotten that there are additional complications of cirrhosis. These include portopulmonary hypertension, hepatopulmonary syndrome, and hepatorenal syndrome type 2.

Evaluation for esophageal varices
Studies have documented that gastroesophageal varices are present in approximately 40% of patients with Child's A cirrhosis and almost 85% of patients with Child's C classification.[41] The platelet count can be a good predictor of the presence or absence of esophageal varices on upper endoscopy. Specifically, a platelet count of 150,000/mm^3 excludes the presence of medium or large esophageal varices with a sensitivity of 90% and negative predictive value of 99%.[42] According to the American Association for the Study of Liver Disease practice guidelines, "screening endoscopy for the diagnosis of esophageal in gastric varices is recommended when the diagnosis of cirrhosis is made."[43] The American Society for Gastrointestinal Endoscopy recommends screening for esophageal varices in "Patients with cirrhosis and portal hypertension but no prior variceal hemorrhage especially those with platelet counts <140,000/mm^3, or Child's Class B or C."[44]

Surveillance for hepatocellular carcinoma

The incidence of hepatocellular carcinoma (HCC) has been rising in various countries.[45,46] Surveillance for HCC should be routinely performed in patients with a diagnosis of cirrhosis of the liver and in patients with chronic hepatitis B. These patients should be entered into a surveillance program using US every 6- to 12-month intervals.[47]

SUMMARY AND FINAL COMMENTS

In summary, evaluation of abnormal LFTs in the hospitalized patient is similar to that in the outpatient setting but often of a more pressing nature. There are 4 steps in this process. The first is to determine if the abnormal LFTs are associated with the major reason for the admission to the hospital or are of chronic nature. The second is to determine the etiology. The third part of this process is to evaluate the severity of the dysfunction and determine if ALF or acute decompensation of chronic liver failure is present. The fourth and final step is to look for associated complications of either acute or chronic liver failure as appropriate. The recommendations section of the consultation form should highlight any missing diagnostic testing for the cause of the disease and the severity of the dysfunction. In addition, there should be clear management guidelines for treatment of the liver disease, the associated complications, as well as a comment regarding the prognosis for the disease and expected response to therapy. A consultation report that focuses on these issues and their management in the best way will provide the most information and value in the evaluation of abnormal LFTs in the hospitalized patient.

REFERENCES

1. Pratt DS, Kaplan MM. Laboratory tests. In: Schiff ER, Sorrell MF, Maddrey WC, editors. 10th edition, Schiff 's diseases of the liver, vol 1. Philadelphia: Lippincott–Raven; 2007. p. 19–60.
2. Nakano T, Shimanuki T, Matsushita M, et al. Involvement of intestinal alkaline phosphatase in serum apolipoprotein B-48 level and its association with ABO and secretor blood group types. Biochem Biophys Res Commun 2006;341(1):33–8.
3. Litin SC, O'Brien JF, Pruett S, et al. Macroenzyme as a cause of unexplained elevation of aspartate aminotransferase. Mayo Clin Proc 1987;62(6):681–7.
4. Begum T, Oliver MR, Kornberg AJ, et al. Elevated aminotransferase as a presenting finding in a patient with occult muscle disease. J Paediatr Child Health 2000; 36(2):189–90.
5. Pratt DS, Kaplan MM. Evaluation of abnormal liver-enzyme results in asymptomatic patients. N Engl J Med 2000;342(17):1267–71.
6. Reichling JJ, Kaplan MM. Clinical use of serum enzymes in liver disease. Dig Dis Sci 1988;33(12):1601–14.
7. Nyblom H, Berggren U, Balldin J, et al. High AST/ALT ratio may indicate advanced alcoholic liver disease rather than heavy drinking. Alcohol 2004; 39(4):336–9.
8. McGarrity TJ, Samuels T, Wilson FA. An analysis of imaging studies and liver function tests to detect hepatic neoplasia. Dig Dis Sci 1987;32(10):1113–7.
9. Pedersen OM, Nordgard K, Kvinnsland S. Value of sonography in obstructive jaundice. Limitations of bile duct caliber as an index of obstruction. Scand J Gastroenterol 1987;22(8):975–81.
10. Pasanen PA, Partanen KP, Pikkarainen PH, et al. A comparison of ultrasound, computed tomography and endoscopic retrograde cholangiopancreatography

in the differential diagnosis of benign and malignant jaundice and cholestasis. Eur J Surg 1993;159(1):23–9.

11. Annet L, Materne R, Danse E, et al. Hepatic flow parameters measured with MR imaging and Doppler US: correlations with degree of cirrhosis and portal hypertension. Radiology 2003;229(2):409–14.

12. Chatziioannou SN, Moore WH, Ford PV, et al. Hepatobiliary scintigraphy is superior to abdominal ultrasonography in suspected acute cholecystitis. Surgery 2000;127(6):609–13.

13. Hoefs JC, Wang F, Kanel G, et al. The liver-spleen scan as a quantitative liver function test: correlation with liver severity at peritoneoscopy. Hepatology 1995; 22(4 Pt 1):1113–21.

14. Zuckerman E, Lobodin G, Sabo E, et al. Quantitative liver-spleen scan using single photon emission computerized tomography (SPECT) for assessment of hepatic function in cirrhotic patients. J Hepatol 2003;39(3):326–32.

15. Rosch T, Meining A, Fruhmorgen S, et al. A prospective comparison of the diagnostic accuracy of ERCP, MRCP, CT, and EUS in biliary strictures. Gastrointest Endosc 2002;55(7):870–6.

16. Bruno MJ. Endoscopic ultrasonography. Endoscopy 2006;38(11):1098–105.

17. Mallery JS, Baron TH, Dominitz JA, et al. Complications of ERCP. Gastrointest Endosc 2003;57(6):633–8.

18. Anciaux ML, Pelletier G, Attali P, et al. Prospective study of clinical and biochemical features of symptomatic choledocholithiasis. Dig Dis Sci 1986;31(5):449–53.

19. Anonymous. NIH state-of-the-science statement on endoscopic retrograde cholangiopancreatography (ERCP) for diagnosis and therapy. NIH Consens State Sci Statements 2002;19(1):1–26.

20. O'Brien CB. Acute and chronic viral hepatitis. In: Rakel RE, Bope ET, editors. Conn's current therapy 2007. Philadelphia: Elsevier Inc; 2007. p. 622–31.

21. Zheng ZB, Wu YD, Yu XL, et al. DNA microarray technology for simultaneous detection and species identification of seven human herpes viruses. J Med Virol 2008;80(6):1042–50.

22. Forget EJ, Menzies D. Adverse reactions to first-line antituberculosis drugs. Expert Opin Drug Saf 2006;5(2):231–49.

23. Kaplowitz N. Causality assessment versus guilt-by-association in drug hepatotoxicity. Hepatology 2001;33(1):308–10.

24. Ostapowicz G, Fontana RJ, Schiodt FV, et al. Results of a prospective study of acute liver failure at 17 tertiary care centers in the United States. Ann Intern Med 2002;137(12):947–54.

25. Knowles SR, Uetrecht J, Shear NH. Idiosyncratic drug reactions: the reactive metabolite syndromes. Lancet 2000;356(9241):1587–91.

26. Andrade RJ, Camargo R, Lucena MI, et al. Causality assessment in drug-induced hepatotoxicity. Expert Opin Drug Saf 2004;3(4):329–44.

27. Johnson RD, O'Connor ML, Kerr RM. Extreme serum elevations of aspartate aminotransferase. Am J Gastroenterol 1995;90(8):1244–5.

28. Seeto RK, Fenn B, Rockey DC. Ischemic hepatitis: clinical presentation and pathogenesis. Am J Med 2000;109(2):109–13.

29. Cohen JA, Kaplan MM. The SGOT/SGPT ratio - an indicator of alcoholic liver disease. Dig Dis Sci 1979;24(11):835–8.

30. Bortolotti F, De Paoli G, Tagliaro F. Carbohydrate-deficient transferrin (CDT) as a marker of alcohol abuse: a critical review of the literature 2001–2005. J Chromatogr B Analyt Technol Biomed Life Sci 2006;841(1–2):96–109.

31. LaMont JT, Isselbacher KJ. Current concepts of postoperative hepatic dysfunction. Conn Med 1975;39(8):461–4.
32. Faust TW, Reddy KR. Postoperative jaundice. Clin Liver Dis 2004;8(1):151–66.
33. Clark JM, Brancati FL, Diehl AM. The prevalence and etiology of elevated aminotransferase levels in the United States. Am J Gastroenterol 2003;98(5):960–7.
34. O'Grady J, Alexander G, Hayllar K, et al. Early indicators of prognosis in fulminant hepatic failure. Gastroenterology 1989;97(2):439–45.
35. Anand AC, Nightingale P, Neuberger JM. Early indicators of prognosis in fulminant hepatic failure: an assessment of the King's criteria. J Hepatol 1997;26(1): 62–8.
36. Mansour A, Watson W, Shayani V, et al. Abdominal operations in patients with cirrhosis: still a major surgical challenge. Surgery 1997;122(4):730–5.
37. Malinchoc M, Kamath PS, Gordon FD, et al. A model to predict poor survival in patients undergoing transjugular intrahepatic portosystemic shunts. Hepatology 2000;31(4):864–71.
38. Kremers WK, van IJperen M, Kim RW, et al. MELD score as a predictor of pre and post transplant survival in OPTN/UNOS status 1 patients. Hepatology 2004;39(4): 764–9.
39. Farnsworth N, Fagan S, Berger D, et al. Child-Turcotte-Pugh versus MELD score as a predictor of outcome after elective and emergent surgery in cirrhotic patients. Am J Surg 2004;188(5):580–3.
40. Rolando N, Harvey F, Brahm J, et al. Prospective study of bacterial infection in acute liver failure: an analysis of fifty patients. Hepatology 1990;11(1):49–53.
41. Pagliaro L, D'Amico G, Pasta L, et al. Portal hypertension in cirrhosis: natural history. In: Bosch J, Groszmann RJ, editors. Portal hypertension, pathophysiology and treatment. Oxford (UK): Blackwell Scientific; 1994. p. 72–92.
42. Sanyal AJ, Fontana RJ, Di Bisceglie AM, et al. The prevalence and risk factors associated with esophageal varices in subjects with hepatitis C and advanced fibrosis. Gastrointest Endosc 2006;64(6):855–64.
43. Garcia-Tsao G, Sanyal AJ, Grace ND, et al. Prevention and management of gastroesophageal varices and variceal hemorrhage in cirrhosis. Hepatology 2007;46(6):922–38.
44. American Society for Gastrointestinal Endoscopy. ASGE guideline: the role of endoscopy in the management of variceal hemorrhage, updated July 2005. Gastrointest Endosc 2005;62(5):651–5.
45. El Serag HB, Mason AC. Rising incidence of hepatocellular carcinoma in the United States. N Engl J Med 1999;340(10):745–50.
46. Parkin DM, Bray F, Ferlay J, et al. Estimating the world cancer burden: Globocan 2000. Int J Cancer 2001;94(2):153–6.
47. Sherman M, Bruix J. AASLD practice guidelines: management of hepatocellular carcinoma. Hepatology 2005;42(5):1208–36.

Approach to a Liver Mass

Oren Shaked, K. Rajender Reddy, MD*

KEYWORDS

- Benign liver mass • Diagnostic tools • Hemangioma
- FNH • NRH • Adenoma • Simple cyst • Cystadenoma

Advances in technology and the widespread use of imaging studies have led to increased detection of liver masses. Often, these masses are discovered incidentally in scans performed for the diagnosis of remotely related or unrelated medical complaints or conditions. Most incidentally discovered masses are benign, requiring little or no medical intervention; however, a conclusive diagnosis must be ascertained to provide patient reassurance. Although it would appear that the most absolute method of identifying a hepatic lesion may be biopsy or pathologic examination of a resected specimen, the increased sensitivity of imaging techniques and the increasing experience among radiologists in interpreting these studies largely mitigate the need for this relatively high-risk procedure. This article is concerned with the selection of the most appropriate diagnostic tools required to determine the nature of the most commonly encountered incidental liver masses (**Tables 1** and **2**).

SOLID LESIONS OF THE LIVER
Hemangioma

Cavernous hemangioma is the most common benign tumor of the liver. Autopsy studies have demonstrated a prevalence of these lesions in the general population ranging from 1.4% to 20%.[1–3] These benign tumors are most often found in women, with a female to male ratio of 2 to 6:1 between the ages of 30 and 50 years, but they are not limited to this age group.[1,4,5] In addition to a higher prevalence, hemangiomas discovered in women tend to be both larger and multiple.[1] Hepatic hemangiomas are multiple in approximately 10% to 33% of cases[1,6,7] and are usually found in the right lobe of the liver.[8,9] The size of these lesions varies widely, with the smallest being only a few millimeters and the largest more than 20 cm. They are most often discovered incidentally (approximately 85% of cases) and are rarely symptomatic.[10] Hemangiomas larger than 4 cm have been defined as giant hemangiomas, and some reports suggest that they are more often associated with clinical implications.[5,11]

School of Medicine, 2 Dulles, 3400 Spruce Street, Hospital of the University of Pennsylvania, Philadelphia, PA 19104, USA
* Corresponding author.
E-mail address: rajender.reddy@uphs.upenn.edu (K.R. Reddy).

Clin Liver Dis 13 (2009) 193–210
doi:10.1016/j.cld.2009.02.004
1089-3261/09/$ – see front matter © 2009 Elsevier Inc. All rights reserved.

liver.theclinics.com

Table 1
Typical presentation of common benign masses

		Hemangioma	FNH	NRH	Adenoma	Simple Cyst	Cystadenoma
Mean age range (y)		30–50	20–40	All ages	All ages	50–70	40–60
Sex ratio (F:M)		2–6:1	8:1	1:1	F>>M	1.5–6:1	4:1
Estrogen sensitive		Possibly	Possibly	No	Yes (causally related)	No	No
US		Hyperechoic	Isoechoic	Isoechoic/ hyperechoic	Hyperechoic	Anechoic with smooth margins	Anechoic with internal septations
CT		Strongly enhances	Central scar	Nonenhancing nodules	Capsule	Isodense to water	Isodense to water
MRI	T1	Hypointense	Isointense/slightly hypointense	Hyperintense nodules	Varied	Hypointense	Hypointense
	T2	Hyperintense	Isointense/slightly hyperintense	Varied nodules	Varied	Hyperintense	Hyperintense

Abbreviations: CT, Computed tomography; FNH, Focal nodular hyperplasia; MRI, Magnetic resonance imaging; NRH, Nodular regenerative hyperplasia; US, Ultrasonography.

Table 2
Frequent questions and strategies in approach to "Incidentaloma"

Tumor Type	Biopsy	Follow-up	OC Use	Pregnancy	Management
Hemangioma	No	Classic features—no follow-up	Not absolutely contraindicated	Not contraindicated	Resect if symptomatic
FNH	No	Classic features—no follow-up	Not absolutely contraindicated	Not contraindicated	Resect if symptomatic
NRH[a]	Yes	Yes—determine underlying disease	Not contraindicated	Not contraindicated	Treat underlying condition. Manage portal hypertension
Adenoma	No	Variable	Discontinue	Generally no (can be individualized)	Resect if solitary and large. Alternatives—embolization ± resection
Simple cyst	No	Observe	Not contraindicated	Not contraindicated	Laparoscopic unroofing if symptomatic. Resection rarely needed
Cystadenoma	No	Investigate surgical options	Not contraindicated	Not contraindicated	Resect

Abbreviation: OC, Oral contraceptive.
[a] May not be encountered as an "incidental" abnormality and is a diffuse process usually as opposed to focality with other lesions.

The etiology of hepatic hemangiomas is unclear. Most consider these lesions to be congenital hamartomas of mesenchymal origin.[5] Histologically, hemangiomas are composed of large vascular spaces that are lined by endothelium and separated by fibrous septa—most likely a result of ectasia rather than neoplastic growth. There is a suggestion that these hepatic masses are influenced by hormonal fluctuations. Estrogen receptors have been exhibited by some but not all cavernous hemangiomas, and reports have indicated that pregnancy and the use of oral contraceptives (OCs) can promote the growth of these lesions.[12–14] Less commonly, hemangiomas can present in men, in women with no history of OC use, and in postmenopausal women, suggesting that hormonal influences are not a precondition for tumor development.[15]

Hemangiomas are asymptomatic in most cases and are discovered incidentally during abdominal imaging for unrelated issues. When symptomatic, the most common manifestation is upper right abdominal pain.[3,5] Other symptoms include nausea, vomiting, and early satiety. Less common presentations include obstructive jaundice, gastric outlet obstruction, hemobilia, inflammatory pseudotumor, caval compression, portal hypertension, and cystic degeneration.[3,5] Symptoms may result from pressure effects on adjacent organs or distension of Glisson's capsule due to tumor size, intra-lesional hemorrhage, localized thrombosis, or torsion of a pedunculated hemangioma; however, symptoms may persist after surgical resection of the hemangioma, indicating that the presumptive relationship between these lesions and pain is not absolute. Disseminated intravascular coagulation in giant hemangiomas, secondary to consumptive coagulopathy, is a rare complication known as Kasabach-Merritt syndrome (KMS), which is seen more often in children and may be precipitated by a surgical or dental procedure.[3]

Hepatic biochemical tests are generally normal, with the exception of cases complicated by KMS or obstructive jaundice. Imaging techniques play a vital role in the accurate diagnosis of these lesions. Most hemangiomas are discovered during sonographic imaging of the abdomen. On conventional ultrasonography (US), hemangiomas typically present as a hyperechoic mass with a well-defined rim and with few intranodular vessels;[16–19] however, sensitivity and specificity are low, ranging from 60% to 75% and 60% to 80%, respectively.[3,20,21] Consequently, US should be reserved for follow-up rather than the diagnosis of hemangioma. New techniques using contrast-enhanced US have significantly increased the sensitivity and specificity of this imaging modality for detecting hemangioma. Reported values for sensitivity range from 76.5% to 92.9% and specificity from 99.4% to 100%.[18,22–24]

Contrast-enhanced dynamic computed tomography (CT) and magnetic resonance imaging (MRI) are both highly specific and sensitive in the detection and diagnosis of hemangioma and should, therefore, be used to make conclusive diagnoses (**Figs. 1** and **2**). The use of standard CT is suboptimal, because the lesion can appear isodense to the liver depending on the phase of the contrast agent. On dynamic CT, hemangiomas show peripheral globular enhancements that are isoattenuating to the aorta with progressive filling in a centripetal fashion.[16,17,25,26] The sensitivity and specificity of this imaging modality are 75% to 85% and 75% to 90%, respectively.[3,27] Hemangiomas are typically hypointense on T1-weighted MRI and hyperintense on T2-weighted images.[16,17,28] They generally appear spherical or ovoid with sharply defined margins.[8] These characteristic findings result in 85% to 96% sensitivity and 85% to 95% specificity when MRI is employed.[3,8,29–31] Planar and single-photon emission CT (SPECT) using technetium-99 m (Tc-99 m)-labeled red blood cells has been shown to increase both the sensitivity and specificity for detection of hemangioma to similar levels achieved by MRI.[7,32] Although less expensive than MRI, this technique fails to detect lesions close to the heart or intrahepatic vessels and tumors smaller than 3 cm.

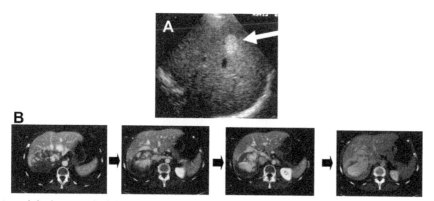

Fig. 1. (*A*) Ultrasound of the liver demonstrating an echodense lesion (*arrow*) consistent with hemangioma. (*B*) CT scan demonstrates a lesion that fills in centripetally on delayed contrast images.

In rare cases, the noninvasive imaging modalities noted here may fail to definitively diagnose hemangiomas. In such instances, angiography may be helpful. Due to the slow blood flow characteristic of hemangioma, these lesions typically have a cotton-wool appearance caused by diffuse pooling of contrast material.[22] In clinical practice, however, rarely is angiography required, and follow-up and demonstration of

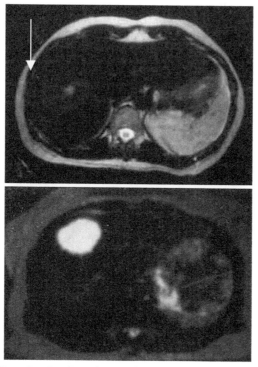

Fig. 2. MRI of the liver showing hyperintense lesion (*arrow*) on T2 image consistent with hemangioma.

stability of the size of the lesion will lend to the diagnostic reliability. Although intuitively it may appear that a biopsy would yield a diagnosis, it has to be kept in mind that there are risks involved with this procedure. Due to the ectatic nature of the lesion, rupture and hemorrhage can be induced by the procedure. In addition, the paucity of reliable histologic characteristics on a needle biopsy necessitates larger core biopsies to make an accurate diagnosis, further increasing the risk of bleeding.

Treatment is rarely indicated for hepatic hemangioma, as most tumors remain asymptomatic and stable over time. It has been suggested that hemangiomas larger than 15 cm may present an increased risk of spontaneous rupture or rupture due to traumatic events, although such events are rare. Surgical resection for the prevention of rare complications does not appear justified. Reports have shown that, when possible, enucleation results in fewer postoperative complications compared with those in resection when dealing with hemangiomas.[4] There have been some reports of radiofrequency ablations and cryoablation of hepatic hemangiomas with good results.[33–35] Liver transplantation is rarely indicated for these benign tumors.

Focal Nodular Hyperplasia

Focal nodular hyperplasia (FNH) is the second most common benign hepatic tumor, with an incidence in the general population ranging from 2.5% to 8%.[36] Most of these lesions are found in women between the ages of 30 and 50 years, with a female to male ratio of 8:1.[37] FNH presents as a single lesion in approximately 80% of the population[37] and is asymptomatic in most cases. These lesions typically range between 3 and 5 cm in size but have been reported as measuring anywhere from 1 mm to 19 cm.[37]

FNH is thought to be the outcome of a congenital vascular malformation, causing normal hepatic parenchyma to form a central scar that radiates out into distinct nodules.[38] Because of its higher prevalence in women, the etiology of these tumors has been assumed to be associated with the use of OCs. However, comparison of the incidence rates of FNH before and after the introduction of OC suggests that the use of OC is not associated with the development of these tumors. Some investigators have suggested that FNH tends to be larger and more vascular in women taking OC;[39] however, one study also demonstrated that there was no correlation between the size of FNH lesions and the length of OC use.[40] These data suggest that there is no causal relationship between the use of OCs and the development of FNH; however, there is some suggestion that these lesions may grow on OCs. However, the recommendation to discontinue OCs is controversial. A reasonable approach, therefore, in those who wish to continue using OCs with a background of FNH would be yearly ultrasound studies to ascertain whether any changes have occurred in the tumor. In contrast, in patients with a firm diagnosis of FNH and no history of OC use, follow-up imaging studies are not recommended.

The clinical manifestations of FNH are few and nonspecific. Most patients are asymptomatic, and lesions are discovered incidentally during abdominal imaging. Approximately 20% to 30% of patients do present with clinical symptoms—most often abdominal pain—leading to the discovery of FNH.[41] Rarely, a palpable mass may be discerned in patients who suffer from large tumors, and hepatomegaly is also sometimes encountered. Patients with FNH generally have normal hepatic biochemical tests.

Differentiating FNH from hepatocellular carcinoma (HCC) and hepatic adenoma is vital. Thus, imaging studies are necessary to make accurate and noninvasive diagnoses of these tumors. FNH is not easily discerned using US, because it generally appears as an isoechoic mass.[5,10,42] The characteristic central scar can be seen as a hyperechoic band in only 20% of cases.[3,43] Sensitivity and specificity are markedly increased when contrast-enhanced US is employed. Using this technique, FNH has a spoked-wheel pattern of blood vessels radiating outward from the central scar.[18,22] Triple-phase CT is considered the best imaging modality for the diagnosis of FNH because of its characteristic attenuating pattern. In the noncontrast phase, the lesion typically presents as an isodense mass, although some variation may be noted.[5,44] The lesion then appears hyperdense in the arterial phase due to its arterial blood supply, and the presence of a central scar is considered the key diagnostic finding in FNH.[42] In the portal venous phase, the lesion again appears isodense due to washout of the contrast agent. In this phase, the central scar may continue to appear hyperattenuating compared with the surrounding tissue. Calcification is not typical in FNH but may be noted in approximately 1% of cases, and so if it is present, a diagnosis other than FNH should be considered.[45,46]

MRI can also be used to diagnose FNH; however, due to its expense and the specificity of CT, it is necessary only for cases in which a diagnosis cannot be determined from other imaging modalities. MRI can detect the central scar of FNH in up to 78% of cases.[47] On T1-weighted images, these lesions appear isointense or slightly hypointense to normal hepatic parenchyma. FNH becomes slightly hyperintense or isointense on T2-weighted images. The use of gadobenate dimeglumine, a hepatic contrast agent, can significantly increase the specificity of MRI for the detection of FNH.[48] The high number of Kupffer cells in these tumors suggests that FNH should readily take up colloid; however, in practice, many FNH lesions do not take up Tc-99 m sulfur colloid, and so these studies cannot be used as a reliable diagnostic tool.

The differentiation of FNH from other benign hepatic lesions is a critical step in the correct management of these tumors. A biopsy is rarely needed when combination-imaging techniques are available; further, needle biopsies are not sufficient to make a diagnosis. Larger, open biopsies are required, putting the patient at increased surgical risk.[10] FNH is rarely symptomatic and does not require medical intervention in most cases. Hemorrhage has been reported in rare cases of FNH;[49] however, there have been no reports of malignant transformations of these benign tumors. Surgery should be undertaken to excise the tumor only in rare cases of severe symptoms or an inconclusive diagnosis.

Nodular Regenerative Hyperplasia

Nodular regenerative hyperplasia (NRH) is a relatively infrequent benign hepatic condition. Autopsy studies have found a 2.6% prevalence of NRH in the general population;[50,51] however, it should be noted that this disorder is commonly associated with other diseases, which may lead to a higher prevalence in an autopsy series. NRH is characterized by a diffuse proliferative process in which normal hepatic parenchyma is replaced by regenerative nodules composed of hyperplastic hepatocytes.[5,10] Each nodule ranges in size from 0.1 to 1 cm.[52] Although NRH is most often found in older patients, it can develop in all age groups. Again, the predominance of NRH in older patients is likely reflective of the association of NRH with other diseases. NRH affects men and women equally, with no identifiable gender predilection.[50,51]

Two theories have been proposed for the development of NRH. The vascular theory describes NRH as a condition resulting from an obstruction in the portal venous system.[52,53] The obstruction leads to thrombosis, causing ischemia and subsequent atrophy of the hepatocytes in zone III. Hepatocytes from the portal region proliferate to compensate for the atrophied cells, thus forming the regenerative nodules. These regenerating nodules compress intrahepatic portal radicles, which may lead to portal hypertension.[3,5] The alternate theory postulates that NRH results because of a generalized proliferative disorder of the liver.[3,54] This theory is supported by the diffusion of dysplastic proliferative nodules throughout the entire liver.

NRH is associated with many diseases and conditions whose presence may help in the diagnosis of this benign disorder. The etiologic correlates that have been linked to NRH are lymphoproliferative disorders, rheumatoid arthritis, primary biliary cirrhosis, bone marrow transplantation, partial hepatectomy, anabolic steroids, hereditary hemorrhagic telangiectasia, polyarteritis nodosa, Budd-Chiari syndrome, liver and renal transplantation, toxic oil exposure, amyloidosis, Felty's syndrome, and HCC.[3,5,10,41,52] Most cases of NRH are asymptomatic[50,51] and are discovered incidentally during evaluation for associated diseases. Patients who are symptomatic present with portal hypertension with ascites and esophageal varices.[52] NRH has also been noted to cause liver failure, necessitating liver transplantation in rare cases. Hepatic biochemical tests are generally normal or slightly elevated; however, fluctuations are nonspecific and, therefore, do not aid in the diagnosis of NRH.[3,5] Patients most commonly present with hepatosplenomegaly during clinical examination.

The radiological features of NRH are not specific enough to make a definitive diagnosis. On ultrasound, the nodules are isoechoic or hyperechoic to normal liver.[5] CT scans present NRH as nonenhancing, hypodense nodules of varying size. Some nodules may appear hyperdense, indicating focal areas of hemorrhage.[55] It can be difficult to distinguish the nodules of NRH from the regenerative nodules of cirrhosis using CT.[3] MRI studies of NRH vary, with nodules usually appearing hyperintense on T1-weighted images and either isointense, slightly hypointense, or hyperintense on T2-weighted images.[56] The presence of Kupffer cells in the regenerative nodules can lead to uptake of Tc-99 m sulfur colloid. Due to the diffuse nature of these lesions, if uptake occurs, scintigraphic images will appear diffuse and patchy. In order to make a definitive diagnosis, more aggressive diagnostic tools are unavoidable. The hepatic histologic abnormalities associated with NRH are more easily observed on gross examination, and, therefore, fine-needle biopsy may not be sufficient in making a diagnosis. NRH and micronodular cirrhosis are similar in appearance, but a diagnosis of NRH can be established based on 3 histologic features: regenerating hepatocytes, curvilinear compression of the central lobule, and a lack of fibrous tissue or fibrous scars between nodules are all indicative of NRH.[3,5,57] Open or laparoscopic biopsies in which a larger tissue sample may be obtained should be reserved for cases in which core or wedge biopsies are unrevealing.

Treatment of NRH depends on the nature of the underlying disease, severity of associated portal hypertension, and symptoms arising from NRH. In most cases, management of the underlying medical condition is sufficient. Patients who suffer from variceal hemorrhage may require recurrent endoscopic therapy or a surgically or radiologically created portosystemic shunt.[3] Transjugular intrahepatic portosystemic shunts (TIPS) are effective in controlling acute variceal bleeding in more than 80% of cases, with a re-bleeding rate of just 18% in patients with underlying liver disease.[58,59] Due to its many drawbacks, including cost, risk of portal systemic encephalopathy, and the need for postprocedural follow-up, TIPS treatment is reserved for severe cases of variceal bleeding in which other modes of therapy have previously been attempted and failed.[58,60] The 5- and 30-year survival rates in NRH cases complicated by portal hypertension are 90% and 55%, respectively, reflecting the absence of associated hepatocellular dysfunction.[61] In rare cases, however, NRH can lead to liver failure, requiring liver transplantation.

Hepatic Adenoma

Hepatic adenomas are relatively rare benign vascular lesions, although they have become more prevalent since the introduction of OCs in the 1960s. These benign proliferations are more often found in young to middle aged women,[62,63] with an incidence of approximately 1 to 1.3 per million in women with no history of OC use and 34 per million in women with long-term exposure to OCs.[5] Lesions are discovered incidentally in about half the patients[63] and are solitary in 71% of patients.[3] Hepatic adenomas are generally found in the right hepatic lobe (66%) and are typically between 5 and 10 cm in diameter,[28] although they have been reported to be larger than 10 cm in about one-third of the cases.[64]

There is a strong relationship between long-term OC use and the development of hepatic adenomas,[65] but a reduction in the dosage of OCs in modern use has lowered the incidence of adenomas in patients on estrogen therapy.[5] The incidence of hepatic adenoma is also higher in patients using androgens[66] as well as patients with underlying metabolic diseases, such as glycogen storage disease types I and III and diabetes mellitus.[36,67] Although the pathogenesis of hepatic adenomas has not been fully elucidated, evidence suggests that these lesions are derived from a single clone of hepatocytes.[68] Expression of the membrane glycoprotein cadherin is greater in the hepatocytes of hepatic adenoma.[69] Cadherin mediates calcium-dependent cell-to-cell adhesions, and its altered expression may play a key role in the development of these benign proliferations. Hepatic adenomas have been broadly categorized into 3 molecular pathologic subgroups: hepatocyte nuclear factor 1α (HNF-1α)-inactivated, β-catenin activated, and inflammatory.[70] Although HNF-1α-inactivated hepatic adenomas have a lower risk of malignant transformation,[71] activated β-catenin mutations can be found in up to 40% of HCCs, suggesting that activation of this gene may increase the tumors' malignant potential.[72]

Many patients with hepatic adenoma are symptomatic. Chronic upper right quadrant or epigastric pain is the most common symptom, although many patients present with severe and sudden pain, which may indicate hemorrhage within the tumor or freely into the peritoneum. Hemodynamic instability and shock state may evolve in those with free intraperitoneal bleeding. Hepatomegaly is another common clinical presentation. The risk of hemorrhage is positively correlated to the size of the tumor, the number of lesions, and a subcapsular location.[5] Symptomatic flares during menstruation have been reported.[73] Hepatic biochemical tests are usually normal.

One of the difficulties encountered in diagnosing and treating hepatic adenoma is its nonspecific appearance on imaging studies. On ultrasound, these lesions appear as well-demarcated masses that are generally hyperechoic because of the high fat content of adenomatous hepatocytes.[10] Increased echogenicity indicates internal hemorrhage, whereas decreased echogenicity is a sign of previous hemorrhage. On noncontrast-enhanced CT, hepatic adenomas tend to be hypodense due to the presence of fat.[64] In contrast, hemorrhagic lesions tend to appear hyperdense. MRIs of hepatic adenomas are variable as well depending on the internal nature of the lesion.[10,28] On T1-weighted images, internal fat and acute hemorrhage increase signal intensity; necrosis, calcification, and past hemorrhage all decrease signal intensity.[74] T2-weighted images are similarly heterogeneous. A recent study has shown that it may be possible to distinguish between the 3 subgroups of hepatocellular adenoma using MRI.[71] HNF-1α-inactivated tumors demonstrate homogenous signal dropout on chemical shift images and only moderate arterial enhancement compared with that of inflammatory hepatic adenomas.[71] In contrast, inflammatory tumors were found to be hyperintense on T2-weighted images, with strong arterial enhancement as well as persistent enhancement in the delayed phase.[71] The study also presented limited evidence that β-catenin activation may be discerned by hypointensity of the signal in the delayed phase.[71] The ability to distinguish between the different subgroups of hepatic adenoma is an important tool in the management of these tumors when assessing their malignant potentials. Scintigraphy may be helpful in differentiating hepatic adenoma from FNH. Unlike FNH, most adenomas lack Kupffer cells, and, consequently, Tc-99 m sulfur colloid scintigraphy shows a characteristic focal defect in 80% of these lesions.[75] Biopsy is not indicated in the diagnosis of hepatic adenoma. Due to the vascular nature of these lesions, the risk of rupture is high. Moreover, lesions may have focal areas of malignancy that may be missed during biopsy.[76]

Conservative management of hepatic adenomas entails high risk because of the propensity of these lesions to hemorrhage or undergo malignant transformation. Approximately 10% of these tumors undergo malignant transformation.[77] When compared with the 1% mortality rate associated with surgical resection, removal of the tumor may be the prudent course. Mortality rates increase to 5% to 8% when emergency resection is undertaken due to rupture.[78] An increase in size, a rise in alpha-fetoprotein levels, and mutations in the β-catenin gene are all associated with malignant transformation, and, therefore, if any of these signs are present, surgical resection should be undertaken.[77,79] Patients who take OC should discontinue estrogen therapy immediately. Reports have indicated that hepatic adenomas may regress after 6 months once estrogens are no longer taken.[80] Regression, however, has its own associated risks, as apparently regressed tumors may still undergo malignant transformation. Patients with hepatic adenomas should be advised to undergo surgical resection before pregnancy because of the increased risk of hemorrhage and growth in tumor size.[81] If the position of a hepatic adenoma is a contraindication to resection, pregnancy should be avoided or pursued with a full understanding of the limited, but definite, risk of rupture or growth causing pain. An alternative to initial hepatic resection is embolization, followed by resection. This strategy may be considered in patients with large adenomas that may present a surgical challenge; these lesions may be accessible to surgical resection after the tumor has undergone necrosis and also a decrease in size. Liver transplantation is rarely indicated except in the case of multiple adenomas or glycogen storage disease. In patients with glycogen storage disease, regression of adenomas has been reported with continuous nocturnal feeding, and so this therapy should be considered for such patients.[5,82] It should be noted, however, that liver transplantation has the potential to correct the underlying metabolic defect.

CYSTIC LESIONS OF THE LIVER
Simple Cyst

Simple hepatic cysts affect approximately 1% to 4% of patients[5,83] and are generally discovered incidentally. There is a positive correlation between age and the incidence of these cysts.[84] Hepatic cysts also occur more commonly in women, with a female to male ratio of 1.5 to 6:1.[83–85] Simple cysts are unilocular and are usually found in the right hepatic lobe.[83,85] Simple cysts range in size anywhere from 1 to 30 cm[84,86] and are generally asymptomatic. Approximately a quarter of these lesions have been reported to present with symptoms,[85] which are generally found in women[87] with larger (>5 cm) cysts.[88]

Histologically, simple cysts are composed of an outer layer of dense fibrous tissue containing an inner layer of cuboidal epithelium. It is thought that these lesions arise from abnormal development of intrahepatic bile ducts in utero.[10] Over time, these aberrant ducts slowly enlarge, leading to the higher prevalence of symptomatic lesions later in life. Cysts that become larger than 5 cm have a higher association with symptoms.[88] The most common symptom is upper right quadrant pain.[84] Other common symptoms include epigastric pain, abdominal distention, dyspnea, nausea, and early satiety.[83,85] Upon physical examination, a hepatic mass or hepatomegaly may be detected. Hepatic biochemical tests are usually normal,[83] leaving imaging technology as the primary diagnostic tool.

US is highly sensitive and specific for the diagnosis of simple cysts.[89] On US, simple cysts appear as anechoic, fluid-filled spaces with smooth margins and imperceptible walls.[10,21,84] Due to the high specificity and sensitivity of US in diagnosing hepatic cysts as well as the low cost of the procedure, CT and MRI studies are less commonly employed. On CT, simple cysts appear isodense to water,[83] they are well demarcated, and they do not enhance when contrast is administered because of the lack of vascularity within the cystic cavity (**Fig. 3**).[83] CT is particularly suitable for specifying the spatial location of cystic lesions relative to the rest of the liver[85] and so may be useful in preparation for surgical intervention. The classic appearance of a simple cyst on MRI is hypointense on T1-weighted images and hyperintense on T2-weighted images.[90] Hyperintensity on both T1- and T2-weighted images suggests hemorrhage within the cyst.[10] Given the typical appearances of hepatic cysts using radiographic imaging techniques, aspiration is not required or recommended.

Conservative management of asymptomatic cysts is recommended due to their relatively benign nature. Some complications associated with cystic lesions that should be screened for are infection, neoplasia, and intracystic hemorrhage.[5] Surgical intervention is the preferred mode of treatment for cysts that do present with symptoms. Fine-needle aspiration with the injection of sclerosing solution or alcohol has been associated with a 100% recurrence rate,[91] and, therefore, should not be considered as a long-term treatment option. Laparoscopic unroofing of solitary hepatic cysts has been performed with significantly improved outcomes, with recurrence rates between 0% to 15%,[83] and so this is the procedure of choice when dealing with these lesions. Partial hepatectomy has also been proposed, although such an invasive procedure is not generally called for and is reserved for symptomatic cysts that are otherwise inaccessible to a laparoscopic unroofing procedure.

Biliary Cystadenoma

Biliary cystadenoma, although rare, is the most common type of primary cystic neoplasm of the liver.[92] These lesions are more commonly found in women, with a male to female ratio of about 4:1, and typically present in quadragenarians.[93] The size of cystadenomas ranges from 2 to 28 cm,[5] and 75% are found in the hepatic parenchyma of the right lobe.[93] Histologically, cystadenomas are multilocular lesions comprising 3 layers of tissue. There is an inner epithelial layer composed of mucus-secreting cuboidal or columnar cells. Around this is a middle mesenchymal layer made up of fibroblasts, smooth muscle, adipose tissue, and capillaries, and surrounding these cells is an outer layer of collagen and mixed connective tissue.[3] There is no cellular atypia or stromal invasion.[83] Approximately 75% of patients present with right upper quadrant or epigastric pain.[83] Other symptoms that are less common include dyspepsia, anorexia, nausea, and vomiting.[93] Symptoms are probably the result of pressure from the cystic mass on adjacent viscera. Secondary infection of these lesions may cause some patients to suffer from fever. On physical examination, a palpable mass may be discerned, or hepatomegaly may be observed if the lesions are large.

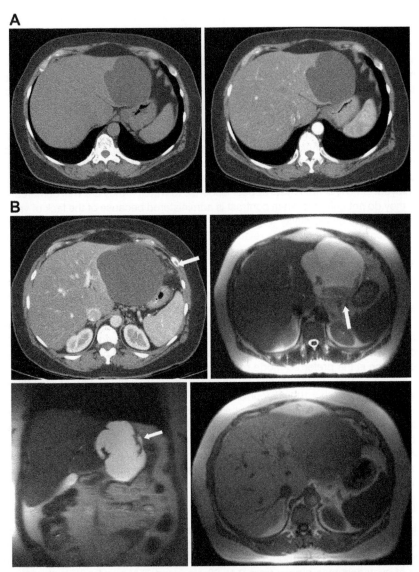

Fig. 3. Hypointense T1 image (*A*) that is hyperintense on T2 image (*B*) consistent with a cyst. Note the irregularity in the border and internally, suggesting that there may have been a bleed (*arrow*). (*Images courtesy of* Claude Sirlin, MD, University of California, San Diego, CA.)

Imaging studies are useful in determining the difference between simple cysts and cystadenomas. Because of the premalignant nature of cystadenoma, it is important to differentiate it from a simple cyst. It has been reported that approximately 25% of cystadenomas undergo malignant transformation to cystadenocarcinoma.[5] On US, these lesions appear as anechoic masses with internal septations and irregular walls;[10] hemorrhagic areas within the lesions present as hyperechoic regions.[94] With CT, cystadenomas appear mostly isoattenuating to water, although there are focal regions that have low attenuation.[95] These regions tend to enhance with the administration of contrast material.[96] Calcification may also be noted within the wall of the cyst.[94,96] MRIs reveal cystadenomas as hypointense on T1-weighted images and hyperintense on T2-weighted images.[97] Treatment of cystadenoma should be aggressive regardless of whether or not symptoms are present in the patient because of the propensity for these lesions to undergo malignant transformation. Resection is the mode of treatment recommended because a complete excision of the cystic lesion markedly reduces the chances of recurrence.[10]

MISCELLANEOUS LESIONS

There are many other types of benign hepatic lesions that may be encountered incidentally, with only the 6 most common having been discussed in this article in detail. Other lesions that must also be considered include liver abscesses, bile duct adenomas, bile duct hamartomas, mesenchymal hamartomas, hemangioendotheliomas, angiomyolipomas, focal fatty infiltrates, inflammatory pseudotumors, macroregenerative nodules, echinococcal cysts, polycystic liver disease, Caroli's disease, traumatic cysts, and ciliated hepatic foregut cysts. HCC must also always be suspected when encountering and diagnosing an incidental hepatic lesion. These tumors have not been covered in this article due to their malignant nature, but they are the most common type of lesions that affect the liver. HCC should be suspected in any patient with a background of chronic viral hepatitis B or C or cirrhosis of any etiology. HCC can occur in hepatitis B infection regardless of the presence or absence of cirrhosis, whereas invariably, in chronic hepatitis C, it is encountered in the background of advanced fibrosis/cirrhosis.

SUMMARY

The incidental discovery of a liver mass has become increasingly common with advancements in imaging technologies, posing many difficulties for physicians. In most cases, these masses are benign and require no medical intervention, a concept not always easily understood by apprehensive patients. The fact is, however, that most people die with a benign liver tumor rather than from one. For this reason, a proper diagnosis is absolutely imperative to provide appropriate patient care.

Many factors must be taken into consideration in the differential diagnosis of liver masses. Gender, age, history of OC use, history of liver disorders, hepatic biochemical tests, and tumor markers can all provide clues that help to identify the type of lesion affecting a patient. When patient characteristics are considered in tandem with high-quality imaging studies, an accurate diagnosis can often be made. If the available information is not conclusive, it is more prudent to employ follow-up imaging than to perform a biopsy to establish an accurate diagnosis. Biopsy is associated with a small, but definite, risk of bleeding. Often, large tissue samples are required to correctly diagnose a benign, solid, hepatic tumor, which can give a false sense of security when a focus of a malignancy in an otherwise benign tumor is missed; therefore, it should be avoided whenever possible.

There are a host of tumors that affect the liver and even more ways in which they can present in patients. This article is concerned with a detailed outline of the 6 most common types of liver masses discovered incidentally during imaging studies for unrelated medical issues. Although the recommendations presented give a general outline for the diagnosis and therapy of these lesions, it is important to always consider the needs of each individual patient. Diagnoses should always be confirmed with the best available imaging tools whenever possible; in most cases, this involves MRI. Benign liver lesions can often be managed conservatively. Surgical options should be reserved only for symptomatic cases or for large adenomas that threaten malignant transformation or have a high risk of bleeding.

REFERENCES

1. Gandolfi L, Leo P, Solmi L, et al. Natural history of hepatic haemangiomas: clinical and ultrasound study. Gut 1991;32(6):677–80.
2. Reddy KR, Kligerman S, Levi J, et al. Benign and solid tumors of the liver: relationship to sex, age, size of tumors, and outcome. Am Surg 2001;67(2):173–8.
3. Trotter JF, Everson GT. Benign focal lesions of the liver. Clin Liver Dis 2001;5(1): 17–42.
4. Gedaly R, Pomposelli JJ, Pomfret EA, et al. Cavernous hemangioma of the liver: anatomic resection vs. enucleation. Arch Surg 1999;134(4):407–11.
5. Karnam US, Reddy KR. Approach to the patient with a liver mass. In: Yamada T, editor. Textbook of gastroenterology. 4th edition. Philadelphia: Lippincott Williams & Wikins; 2003. p. 973–82.
6. Harvey CJ, Albrecht T. Ultrasound of focal liver lesions. Eur Radiol 2001;11(9): 1578–93.
7. Rubin RA, Lichtenstein GR. Scintigraphic evaluation of liver masses: cavernous hepatic hemangioma. J Nucl Med 1993;34(5):849–52.
8. Stark DD, Felder RC, Wittenberg J, et al. Magnetic resonance imaging of cavernous hemangioma of the liver: tissue-specific characterization. Am J Roentgenol 1985;145(2):213–22.
9. Yoon SS, Charny CK, Fong Y, et al. Diagnosis, management, and outcomes of 115 patients with hepatic hemangioma. J Am Coll Surg 2003;197(3):392–402.
10. Mergo PJ, Ros PR. Benign lesions of the liver. Radiol Clin North Am 1998;36(2): 319–31.
11. Adam YG, Huvos AG, Fortner JG. Giant hemangiomas of the liver. Ann Surg 1970;172(2):239–45.
12. Conter RL, Longmire WP Jr. Recurrent hepatic hemangiomas. Possible association with estrogen therapy. Ann Surg 1988;207(2):115–9.
13. Glinkova V, Shevah O, Boaz M, et al. Hepatic haemangiomas: possible association with female sex hormones. Gut 2004;53(9):1352–5.
14. Saegusa T, Ito K, Oba N, et al. Enlargement of multiple cavernous hemangioma of the liver in association with pregnancy. Intern Med 1995;34(3):207–11.
15. Farges O, Daradkeh S, Bismuth H. Cavernous hemangiomas of the liver: are there any indications for resection? World J Surg 1995;19(1):19–24.
16. Bree RL, Schwab RE, Glazer GM, et al. The varied appearances of hepatic cavernous hemangiomas with sonography, computed tomography, magnetic resonance imaging, and scintigraphy. Radiographics 1987;7(6):1153–75.
17. Jang HJ, Kim TK, Lim HK, et al. Hepatic hemangioma: atypical appearances on CT, MR imaging, and sonography. Am J Roentgenol 2003;180(1):135–41.
18. Quaia E, Calliada F, Bertolotto M, et al. Characterization of focal liver lesions with contrast-specific US modes and a sulfur hexafluoride-filled microbubble contrast agent: diagnosis performance and confidence. Radiology 2004;232(2):420–30.
19. Wilson SR, Burns PN, Muradali D, et al. Harmonic hepatic US with microbubble contrast agent: initial experience showing improved characterization of hemangioma, hepatocellular carcinoma, and metastasis. Radiology 2000;215(1): 153–61.
20. Tanaka S, Ioka T, Oshikawa O, et al. Dynamic sonography of hepatic tumors. Am J Roentgenol 2001;177(4):799–805.

21. Marn C, Bree R, Silver T. Ultrasonography of liver. Technique and focal and diffuse disease. Radiol Clin North Am 1991;29(6):1151–70.
22. Wen YL, Kudo M, Zheng RQ, et al. Characterization of hepatic tumors: value of contrast-enhanced coded phase-inversion harmonic angio. Am J Roentgenol 2004;182(4):1019–26.
23. Furuse J, Nagase M, Ishii H, et al. Contrast enhancement patterns of hepatic tumours during the vascular phase using coded harmonic imaging and Levovist to differentiate hepatocellular carcinoma from other focal lesions. Br J Radiol 2003;76(906):385–92.
24. Isozaki T, Numata K, Kiba T, et al. Differential diagnosis of hepatic tumors by using contrast enhancement patterns at US. Radiology 2003;229(3):798–805.
25. Yun EJ, Choi BI, Han JK, et al. Hepatic hemangioma: contrast-enhancement pattern during the arterial and portal venous phases of spiral CT. Abdom Imaging 1999;24(3):262–6.
26. Yamashita Y, Ogata I, Urata J, et al. Cavernous hemangioma of the liver: pathologic correlation with dynamic CT findings. Radiology 1997;203(1):121–5.
27. van Leeuwen MS, Noordzij J, Feldberg MA, et al. Focal liver lesions: characterization with triphasic spiral CT. Radiology 1996;201(2):327–36.
28. Powers C, Ros PR, Stoupis C, et al. Primary liver neoplasms: MR imaging with pathologic correlation. Radiographics 1994;14(3):459–82.
29. Bennett GL, Petersein A, Mayo-Smith WW, et al. Addition of gadolinium chelates to heavily T2-weighted MR imaging: limited role in differentiating hepatic hemangioma from metastases. Am J Roentgenol 2000;174(2):477–85.
30. Kumano S, Murakami T, Kim T, et al. Using superparamagnetic iron oxide-enhanced MRI to differential metastatic hepatic tumors and nonsolid benign lesions. Am J Roentgenol 2003;181(5):1335–9.
31. Soyer P, Gueye C, Somveille E, et al. MR diagnosis of hepatic metastases from neuroendocrine tumors versus hemangiomas: relative merits of dynamic gadolinium chelate-enhanced gradient-recalled echo and unenhanced spin-echo images. Am J Roentgenol 1995;165(6):1407–13.
32. el-Desouki M, Mohamadiyeh M, al-Rashed R, et al. Features of hepatic cavernous hemangioma on planar and SPECT Tc-99m-labeled red blood cell scintigraphy. Clin Nucl Med 1999;24(8):583–9.
33. Hinshaw JL, Laeseke PJ, Weber SM, et al. Multiple-electrode radiofrequency ablation of symptomatic hepatic cavernous hemangioma. Am J Roentgenol 2007;189(3):W146–9.
34. Silverman SG, Tuncali K, Adams DF, et al. MR imaging-guided percutaneous cryotherapy of liver tumors: initial experience. Radiology 2000;217(3):657–64.
35. Zagoria RJ, Roth TJ, Levine EA, et al. Radiofrequency ablation of a symptomatic hepatic cavernous hemangioma. Am J Roentgenol 2004;182(1):210–2.
36. Craig JR, Peters RL, Edmonson HA. Tumors of the liver and intrahepatic bile ducts. In: Hartmann WH, editor. Atlas of tumor pathology, series 2. Washington: Armed Forces Institute of Pathology; 1989. p. 63–101.
37. Nguyen BN, Flejou JF, Terris B, et al. Focal nodular hyperplasia of the liver: a comprehensive pathological study of 305 lesions and recognition of new histologic forms. Am J Surg Pathol 1999;23(12):1441–54.
38. Wanless IR, Mawdsley C, Adams R. On the pathogenesis of focal nodular hyperplasia of the liver. Hepatology 1985;5(6):1194–200.
39. Scalori A, Tavani A, Gallus S, et al. Oral contraceptives and the risk of focal nodular hyperplasia of the liver: a case-control study. Am J Obstet Gynecol 2002;186(2):195–7.

40. Mathieu D, Kobeiter H, Maison P, et al. Oral contraceptive use and focal nodular hyperplasia of the liver. Gastroenterology 2000;118(3):560–4.
41. Blonski W, Reddy KR. Evaluation of nonmalignant liver masses. Curr Gastroenterol Rep 2006;8(1):38–45.
42. Kehagias D, Moulopoulos L, Antoniou A, et al. Focal nodular hyperplasia: imaging findings. Eur Radiol 2001;11(2):202–12.
43. Shamsi K, De Schepper A, Degryse H, et al. Focal nodular hyperplasia of the liver: radiologic findings. Abdom Imaging 1993;18(1):32–8.
44. Carlson SK, Johnson CD, Bender CE, et al. CT of focal nodular hyperplasia of the liver. Am J Roentgenol 2000;174(3):705–12.
45. Caseiro-Alves F, Zins M, Mahfouz A-E, et al. Calcification in focal nodular hyperplasia: a new problem for differentiation from fibrolamellar hepatocellular carcinoma. Radiology 1996;198(3):889–92.
46. Blachar A, Federle MP, Ferris JV, et al. Radiologists' performance in the diagnosis of liver tumors with central scars by using specific CT criteria. Radiology 2002; 223(2):532–9.
47. Cherqui D, Rahmouni A, Charlotte F, et al. Management of focal nodular hyperplasia and hepatocellular adenoma in young women: a series of 41 patients with clinical, radiological, and pathological correlations. Hepatology 1995;22(6):1674–81.
48. Grazioli L, Morana G, Kirchin MA, et al. Accurate differentiation of focal nodular hyperplasia from hepatic adenoma at gadobenate dimeglumine-enhanced MR imaging: prospective study. Radiology 2005;236(1):166–77.
49. Becker CD, Gal I, Baer HU, et al. Blunt hepatic trauma in adults: correlation of CT injury grading with outcome. Radiology 1996;201(1):215–20.
50. Wanless IR. Micronodular transformation (nodular regenerative hyperplasia) of the liver: a report of 64 cases among 2,500 autopsies and a new classification of benign hepatocellular nodules. Hepatology 1990;11(5):787–97.
51. Nakanuma Y. Nodular regenerative hyperplasia of the liver: retrospective survey in autopsy series. J Clin Gastroenterol 1990;12(4):460–5.
52. Reshamwala PA, Kleiner DE, Heller T. Nodular regenerative hyperplasia: not all nodules are created equal. Hepatology 2006;44(1):7–14.
53. Ibarrola C, Colina F. Clinicopathological features of nine cases of non-cirrhotic portal hypertension: current definitions and criteria are inadequate. Histopathology 2003;42(3):251–64.
54. Nzeako UC, Goodman ZD, Ishak KG. Hepatocellular carcinoma and nodular regenerative hyperplasia: possible pathogenetic relationship. Am J Gastroenterol 1996;91(5):879–84.
55. Dachman AH, Ros PR, Goodman ZD, et al. Nodular regenerative hyperplasia of the liver: clinical and radiologic observations. Am J Roentgenol 1987;148(4): 717–22.
56. Rha SE, Lee MG, Lee YS, et al. Nodular regenerative hyperplasia of the liver in Budd-Chiari syndrome: CT and MR features. Abdom Imaging 2000;25(3):255–8.
57. Al-Mukhaizeem KA, Rosenberg A, Sherker AH. Nodular regenerative hyperplasia of the liver: an under-recognized cause of portal hypertension in hematological disorders. Am J Hematol 2004;75(4):225–30.
58. Colombato L. The role of Transjugular Intrahepatic Portosystemic Shunt (TIPS) in the management of portal hypertension. J Clin Gastroenterol 2007;41(S3): S344–51.
59. Boyer TD, Haskal ZJ. American Association for the Study of Liver Diseases. The role of transjugular intrahepatic portosystemic shunt in the management of portal hypertension. Hepatology 2005;41(2):386–400.

60. Boyer TD. Transjugular intrahepatic portosystemic shunt in the management of complications of portal hypertension. Curr Gastroenterol Rep 2008;10(1):30–5.

61. Faust D, Fellbaum C, Zeuzem S, et al. Nodular regenerative hyperplasia of the liver: a rare differential diagnosis of cholestasis with response to ursodeoxycholic acid. Z Gastroenterol 2003;41(3):255–8.

62. Terkivatan T, de Wilt JH, de Man RA, et al. Indications and long-term outcome of treatment for benign hepatic tumors: a critical approach. Arch Surg 2001;136(9): 1033–8.

63. Weinmann A, Ringe B, Klempnauer J, et al. Benign liver tumors: differential diagnosis and indications for surgery. World J Surg 1997;21(9):983–90.

64. Ichikawa T, Federle MP, Grazioli L, et al. Hepatocellular adenoma: multiphasic CT and histopathologic findings in 25 patients. Radiology 2000;214(3):861–8.

65. Edmondson HA, Henderson B, Benton B. Liver-cell adenomas associated with use of oral contraceptives. N Engl J Med 1976;294(9):470–2.

66. Carrasco D, Prieto M, Pallardó L, et al. Multiple hepatic adenomas after long-term therapy with testosterone enanthate. Review of the literature. J Hepatol 1985;1(6):573–8.

67. Labrune P, Trioche P, Duvaltier I, et al. Hepatocellular adenomas in glycogen storage disease type I and III: a series of 43 patients and review of the literature. J Pediatr Gastroenterol Nutr 1997;24(3):276–9.

68. Gaffey MJ, Iezzoni JC, Weiss LM. Clonal analysis of focal nodular hyperplasia of the liver. Am J Pathol 1996;148(4):1089–96.

69. Kozyraki R, Scoazec JY, Flejou JF, et al. Expression of cadherins and α-catenin in primary epithelial tumors of the liver. Gastroenterology 1996;110(4):1137–49.

70. Rebouissou S, Bioulac-Sage P, Zucman-Rossi J. Molecular pathogenesis of focal nodular hyperplasia and hepatocellular adenoma. J Hepatol 2008;48(1):163–70.

71. Laumonier H, Bioulac-Sage P, Laurent C, et al. Hepatocellular adenomas: magnetic resonance imaging features as a function of molecular pathological classification. Hepatology 2008;48(3):808–18.

72. de La Coste A, Romagnolo B, Billuart P, et al. Somatic mutations of the β-catenin gene are frequent in mouse and human hepatocellular carcinomas. Proc Natl Acad Sci U S A 1998;95(15):8847–51.

73. Rooks JB, Ory HW, Ishak KG, et al. Epidemiology of hepatocellular adenoma. The role of oral contraceptive use. JAMA 1979;242(7):644–8.

74. Grazioli L, Federle MP, Brancatelli G, et al. Hepatic adenomas: imaging and pathologic findings. Radiographics 2001;21(4):877–92.

75. Rubin RA, Lichtenstein GR. Hepatic scintigraphy in the evaluation of solitary solid liver masses. J Nucl Med 1993;34(4):697–705.

76. Ferrell LD. Hepatocellular carcinoma arising in a focus of multilobular adenoma. A case report. Am J Surg Pathol 1993;17(5):525–9.

77. Foster JH, Berman MM. The malignant transformation of liver cell adenomas. Arch Surg 1994;129(7):712–7.

78. Krasinskas AM, Eghtesad B, Kamath PS, et al. Liver transplantation for severe intrahepatic noncirrhotic portal hypertension. Liver Transpl 2005;11(6):627–34.

79. Zucman-Rossi J, Jeannot E, Nhieu JT, et al. Genotype-phenotype correlation in hepatocellular adenoma: new classification and relationship with HCC. Hepatology 2006;43(3):515–24.

80. Edmondson HA, Reynolds TB, Henderson B, et al. Regression of liver cell adenomas associated with oral contraceptives. Ann Intern Med 1977;86(2): 180–2.

81. Estebe JP, Malledant Y, Guillou YM, et al. [Spontaneous rupture of an adenoma of the liver during pregnancy]. J Chir (Paris) 1988;125(11):654–6.

82. Parker P, Burr I, Slonim A, et al. Regression of hepatic adenomas in type Ia glycogen storage disease with dietary therapy. Gastroenterology 1981;81(3): 534–6.

83. Regev A, Reddy KR, Berho M, et al. Large cystic lesions of the liver in adults: a 15-year experience in a tertiary center. J Am Coll Surg 2001;193(1):36–45.

84. Nisenbaum HL, Rowling SE. Ultrasound of focal hepatic lesions. Semin Roentgenol 1995;30(4):324–46.

85. Cowles RA, Mulholland MW. Solitary hepatic cysts. J Am Coll Surg 2000;191(3): 311–21.

86. Bahirwani R, Reddy KR. Review article: evaluation of solitary liver masses. Aliment Pharmacol Ther 2008;28:953–65.

87. Martin IJ, McKinley AJ, Currie EJ, et al. Tailoring the management of nonparasitic liver cysts. Ann Surg 1998;228(2):167–72.

88. Taylor BR, Langer B. Current surgical management of hepatic cyst disease. Adv Surg 1997;31:127–48.

89. Spiegel RM, King DL, Green WM. Ultrasonography of primary cysts of the liver. Am J Roentgenol 1978;131(2):235–8.

90. Kanzer GK, Weinreb JC. Magnetic resonance imaging of diseases of the liver and biliary system. Radiol Clin North Am 1991;29(6):1259–84.

91. Saini S, Mueller PR, Ferrucci JT Jr, et al. Percutaneous aspiration of hepatic cysts does not provide definitive therapy. Am J Roentgenol 1983;141(3):559–60.

92. Alobaidi M, Shirkhoda A. Benign focal liver lesions: discrimination from malignant mimickers. Curr Probl Diagn Radiol 2004;33(6):239–53.

93. Ishak KG, Willis GW, Cummins SD, et al. Biliary cystadenoma and cystadenocarcinoma: report of 14 cases and review of the literature. Cancer 1977;39(1): 322–38.

94. Buetow PC, Buck JL, Pantongrag-Brown L, et al. Biliary cystadenoma and cystadenocarcinoma: clinical-imaging-pathologic correlation with emphasis on the importance of ovarian stroma. Radiology 1995;196(3):805–10.

95. Choi BI, Lim JH, Han MC, et al. Biliary cystadenoma and cystadenocarcinoma: CT and sonographic findings. Radiology 1989;171(1):57–61.

96. Korobkin M, Stephens DH, Lee JK, et al. Biliary cystadenoma and cystadenocarcinoma: CT and sonographic findings. Am J Roentgenol 1989;153(3):507–11.

97. Mortelé KJ, Ros PR. Cystic focal liver lesions in the adult: differential CT and MR imaging features. Radiographics 2001;21(4):895–910.

Surgery in the Patient with Liver Disease

Jacqueline G. O'Leary, MD, MPH[a], Patrick S. Yachimski, MD, MPH[b,c,d],
Lawrence S. Friedman, MD[e,f,g,h],*

KEYWORDS

- Cirrhosis • Surgery • MELD score
- Child class • Liver disease

Administration of anesthesia reduces blood flow to the liver during all surgical procedures. In patients with normal liver function, the reduction in blood flow can result in asymptomatic elevation in the results of serum liver biochemical tests postoperatively; in patients with compromised liver function preoperatively, hepatic decompensation can occur intra- and postoperatively, leading to morbidity and mortality. Because liver disease is common and patients with liver disease are frequently asymptomatic, the preoperative assessment of all patients undergoing surgery must include a careful history and physical examination to uncover risk factors for and evidence of liver dysfunction. If liver disease is present, elective surgery should be deferred until the patient has been evaluated or recovered. Operative risk correlates with the severity of the underlying liver disease and the nature of the surgical procedure. In patients with cirrhosis, the Child class and Model for End-Stage liver Disease (MELD) score should be calculated to assist in preoperative risk assessment. When patients with decompensated liver disease must undergo surgery, their clinical condition should be optimized perioperatively to improve the chances of a favorable outcome.

EFFECTS OF ANESTHESIA AND SURGERY ON THE LIVER
Changes in Liver Biochemical Test Levels

Most surgical procedures, whether performed under general or conduction (spinal or epidural) anesthesia, are followed by minor elevations in the results of serum liver

[a] Division of Hepatology, Department of Internal Medicine, Baylor University Medical Center, 4th Floor Roberts, 3500 Gaston Avenue, Dallas, TX 75246, USA
[b] Department of Medicine, Harvard Medical School, Boston, MA 02115, USA
[c] Gastrointestinal Unit, Massachusetts General Hospital, Blake 4, 55 Fruit Street, Boston, MA 02114, USA
[d] Division of Gastroenterology, Brigham and Women's Hospital, Boston, MA 02115, USA
[e] Department of Medicine, Harvard Medical School, Boston, MA 02115, USA
[f] Department of Medicine, Tufts University School of Medicine, Boston, MA 02110, USA
[g] Department of Medicine, Newton-Wellesley Hospital, 2014 Washington Street, Newton, MA 02462, USA
[h] Department of Medicine, Massachusetts General Hospital, Boston, MA 02114, USA
* Corresponding author.
E-mail address: lfriedman@partners.org (L.S. Friedman).

Clin Liver Dis 13 (2009) 211–231
doi:10.1016/j.cld.2009.02.002
1089-3261/09/$ – see front matter © 2009 Elsevier Inc. All rights reserved.

biochemical tests.[1,2] Minor postoperative elevations of serum aminotransferase, alkaline phosphatase, or bilirubin levels in patients without underlying cirrhosis are not clinically significant. However, in patients with underlying liver disease, and especially those with compromised hepatic synthetic function, surgery can precipitate frank hepatic decompensation.

Hemodynamic Effects

Cirrhosis is associated with a hyperdynamic circulation with increased cardiac output and decreased systemic vascular resistance. At baseline, hepatic arterial and venous perfusion of the cirrhotic liver may be decreased: portal blood flow is reduced as a result of portal hypertension, and arterial blood flow can be decreased because of impaired autoregulation. Moreover, patients with cirrhosis may have alterations in the systemic circulation due to arteriovenous shunting and reduced splanchnic inflow. The decreased hepatic perfusion at baseline makes the cirrhotic liver more susceptible to hypoxemia and hypotension in the operating room. Anesthetic agents may reduce hepatic blood flow by 30% to 50% following induction.[2] Animal data suggest, however, that isoflurane (along with desflurane and sevoflurane, which are believed to be similar) causes less perturbation in hepatic arterial blood flow than other inhaled anesthetic agents and therefore is preferred for patients with liver disease.[3]

Additional factors that may contribute to decreased hepatic blood flow intraoperatively include hypotension, hemorrhage, and vasoactive drugs. Intermittent positive-pressure ventilation and pneumoperitoneum during laparoscopic surgery mechanically decrease hepatic blood flow.[4] In addition, traction on the abdominal viscera may cause reflex dilatation of splanchnic capacitance vessels and thereby lower hepatic blood flow.

Hypoxemia

Risk factors for acute intraoperative hypoxemia in patients with cirrhosis include ascites and hepatic hydrothorax. Postoperatively, ascites, encephalopathy, and anesthetic agents increase the risk of pulmonary aspiration in patients with cirrhosis. Hepatopulmonary syndrome (HPS)—the triad of liver disease, an increased alveolar-arterial gradient, and intrapulmonary shunting—is found in 5% to 32% of cirrhotic patients followed at transplant centers.[5] Clues to the presence of HPS include platypnea (increased dyspnea in an upright posture) and orthodeoxia (oxygen desaturation in an upright posture). Portopulmonary hypertension—pulmonary hypertension associated with cirrhosis—is found in up to 6% of patients with advanced liver disease.[6] Although published data regarding surgery in patients with portopulmonary hypertension are limited, pulmonary hypertension regardless of the cause has been shown to increase postoperative mortality after noncardiac surgery.[7]

The severity of HPS and portopulmonary hypertension does not correlate with the severity of associated liver disease. These pulmonary processes must be suspected in any patient with hypoxia and cirrhosis regardless of hepatic synthetic function. In addition, both conditions significantly increase the risk of perioperative mortality. Therefore, elective surgery should be avoided in patients with either HPS or portopulmonary hypertension.

Hepatic Metabolism of Anesthetic Agents and Perioperative Medications

Acute hepatitis associated with the administration of halothane, now rarely used, is believed to be caused by immune sensitization to trifluoroacetylated liver proteins formed by oxidative metabolism of halothane by cytochrome P450 2E1 in genetically predisposed persons.[8] With this notable exception, few data suggest that either the choice of anesthetic agent or mode of administration (inhaled or spinal) influences surgical outcome in patients with liver disease.[9]

In many patients with cirrhosis the volume of distribution of drugs is increased. In addition, the action of anesthetic agents may be prolonged in patients with liver disease because of impaired metabolism and hypoalbuminemia (resulting in decreased drug binding and impaired biliary clearance). Propofol is an excellent anesthetic choice in patients with liver disease, because it retains a short half-life even in patients with decompensated cirrhosis.[10] Unlike halothane, hepatitis caused by isoflurane, desflurane, and sevoflurane, which undergo little hepatic metabolism, is rare. These anesthetic agents are also good choices in patients with liver disease.

The volume of distribution of nondepolarizing muscle relaxants is increased in patients with liver disease, and therefore larger doses may be required to achieve adequate neuromuscular blockade. Atracurium and cisatracurium are the preferred muscle relaxants in patients with liver disease because neither the liver nor the kidney are required for their elimination. Doxacurium is the preferred muscle relaxant in longer procedures such as liver transplantation, as it is metabolized by the kidney.

Sedatives, narcotics, and intravenous induction agents are generally well tolerated in patients with compensated liver disease but must be used with caution in patients with hepatic dysfunction, because they may cause prolonged depression of consciousness and precipitate hepatic encephalopathy. Blood levels of narcotics that undergo high first-pass extraction by the liver increase as hepatic blood flow decreases. Elimination of benzodiazepines that undergo glucuronidation (eg, oxazepam, lorazepam) is unaffected by liver disease, whereas the elimination of those that do not undergo glucuronidation (eg, diazepam, chlordiazepoxide) is prolonged in liver disease. In general, narcotics and benzodiazepines should be avoided in these patients; however, when necessary, remifentanil is the preferred narcotic and oxazepam is the preferred sedative, because the metabolism of these agents is unaffected by liver disease.

OPERATIVE RISK IN PATIENTS WITH LIVER DISEASE
Challenges in Estimating Operative Risk

In a patient with liver disease, surgical risk depends on the degree of hepatic dysfunction, the nature of the surgical procedure, and the presence of comorbid conditions. There are several liver-related contraindications to elective surgery (**Box 1**). When these contraindications are absent, patients with liver disease should undergo a thorough preoperative evaluation, and care of their liver disease should be optimized before elective surgery. Patients found to have advanced liver disease may be best managed with nonsurgical interventions if appropriate.

Once liver disease is identified in a patient who requires surgery, an assessment of the severity of liver disease should be undertaken, as should an evaluation for other nonhepatic risk factors for perioperative mortality (**Box 2**). Data from studies of patients with cirrhosis suggest that the severity of liver disease can best be assessed by the Child–Turcotte–Pugh (CTP) score (Child class) and MELD score (see section on Stratification by MELD score). Additional comorbid conditions increase the morbidity and mortality of surgery in patients with liver disease, although their effects are difficult to quantitate.

Most published studies describing operative risk in patients with liver disease are based on single-center, retrospective cohorts in patients with cirrhosis. These data have limitations, including small cohort size, selection bias, and lack of external validation. Despite these limitations, the results of studies describing operative risk in

---

Box 1
Contraindications to elective surgery in patients with liver disease

Acute liver failure

Acute renal failure

Acute viral hepatitis

Alcoholic hepatitis

Cardiomyopathy

Hypoxemia

Severe coagulopathy (despite treatment)

---

patients with liver disease have been remarkably consistent. As one might expect, operative morbidity and mortality increase with increasing severity of liver disease, as reflected in the Child class or MELD score. In general, patients with compensated cirrhosis who have normal synthetic function have a low overall risk, and the risk increases for patients with decompensated cirrhosis.

Preoperative Screening

Whether healthy, asymptomatic patients should undergo routine preoperative liver biochemical testing is debatable. The prevalence of elevated serum aminotransferases in serum in the adult population in the United States is 9.8%.[11] Not only is the

---

Box 2
Risk factors for surgery in patients with cirrhosis

Patient characteristics

Anemia

Ascites

Child class (Child–Turcotte–Pugh score)

Encephalopathy

Hypoalbuminemia

Hypoxemia

Infection

Malnutrition

MELD score

Portal hypertension

Prolonged prothrombin time (>2.5 seconds) that does not correct with vitamin K

Type of surgery

Cardiac surgery

Emergency surgery

Hepatic resection

Open abdominal surgery

Abbreviation: MELD, Model for End-Stage Liver Disease.

---

presence of an elevated aminotransferase level associated with liver disease but also patients with an elevated serum alanine aminotransferase level in the absence of viral hepatitis or excessive alcohol use may be at increased long-term risk of coronary heart disease and mortality, probably because the alanine aminotransferase level correlates with the presence of metabolic syndrome and its individual components, including obesity and diabetes mellitus.[12]

Reliance on routine liver biochemical tests alone may be misleading, because patients with cirrhosis may have normal results. Therefore, laboratory testing can never replace thorough history taking and physical examination. Obtaining liver biochemical tests preoperatively for screening purposes in asymptomatic persons without risk factors or physical findings indicating liver disease is not routinely recommended preoperatively.

The evaluation should include careful history taking to identify risk factors for liver disease, including prior blood transfusion, illicit drug use, sexual promiscuity, a family history of jaundice or liver disease, a personal history of jaundice, excessive alcohol use, and use of potentially hepatotoxic medications, including over-the-counter and herbal preparations. In some cases, cirrhosis may be suspected after evaluation for characteristic symptoms such as pruritus or fatigue, or on the basis of findings on physical examination such as palmar erythema, spider telangiectasias, abnormal hepatic contour or size, splenomegaly, hepatic encephalopathy, ascites, testicular atrophy, or gynecomastia.

When liver disease is suspected on the basis of physical examination findings or persistent liver biochemical test abnormalities, elective surgery should be deferred so that additional investigations can be undertaken, including biochemical and serologic testing for viral hepatitis, autoimmune liver disease, and metabolic disorders. Abdominal ultrasonography or magnetic resonance cholangiopancreatography may be considered when biliary obstruction is suspected. Abdominal computed tomography or magnetic resonance imaging may reveal a liver size and contour suggestive of cirrhosis or may detect intraabdominal varices and splenomegaly compatible with portal hypertension, but cannot reliably identify hepatic fibrosis or cirrhosis. Although noninvasive serologic and radiologic testing is often adequate for diagnosis and surgical risk assessment, liver biopsy remains the gold standard for the diagnosis and staging of liver disease.

Conditions for which Elective Surgery is Generally Contraindicated

Acute hepatitis

Acute hepatitis may be caused by viruses, drugs, and toxins (including those contained in over-the-counter medications, herbal preparations, and alcohol), autoimmune diseases, and genetic disorders. In addition, hypoperfusion, vascular congestion, and hepatic clotting disorders can lead to acute liver injury without significant inflammation. The cause of acute hepatitis can be determined in most instances noninvasively by history taking, physical examination, imaging, and serologic testing. A liver biopsy is sometimes needed for diagnosis and staging.

Patients with acute hepatitis of any cause are regarded as having an increased operative risk.[2] This conclusion is based on data from older studies, in which operative mortality rates of 10% to 13% were reported among patients who underwent laparotomy to distinguish intrahepatic from extrahepatic causes of jaundice.[13,14]

Although diagnostic and surgical techniques have improved since these studies were published, elective surgery is still contraindicated in patients with acute hepatitis. In most cases, acute hepatitis is either self-limited or treatable, and elective surgery can be undertaken after the patient improves clinically and biochemically.

Alcoholic hepatitis

Alcoholic hepatitis is a contraindication to elective surgery and greatly increases perioperative mortality after urgent or emergency surgery. Fever, right upper quadrant tenderness, and leukocytosis can occur in patients with alcoholic hepatitis, which must be distinguished from acute cholecystitis and ascending cholangitis.[15] Gallbladder wall edema, caused by hypoalbuminemia, can result from alcoholic hepatitis. In addition, hyperbilirubinemia, more often associated with alcoholic hepatitis, greatly impairs the diagnostic accuracy of cholescintigraphy (eg, a hydroxy iminodiacetic acid scan).

Laparotomy performed in a patient with alcoholic hepatitis may have serious consequences.[16] In a retrospective series of patients with alcoholic hepatitis, the mortality rate was 58% among the 12 patients who underwent open liver biopsy, compared with 10% among the 39 who underwent percutaneous liver biopsy. Because only 1 death in the former group was secondary to intraabdominal hemorrhage, open abdominal surgery, rather than liver biopsy, is likely to have been responsible for the high mortality rate.

Abstinence from alcohol for at least 12 weeks generally results in dramatic improvement in hepatic inflammation and hyperbilirubinemia. After more than 12 weeks of abstinence from alcohol, the patient should undergo a thorough reassessment of hepatic function before elective surgery is considered.

Acute liver failure

Patients with acute liver failure (defined as the development of jaundice, coagulopathy, and hepatic encephalopathy within 26 weeks in a patient with acute liver injury in the absence of preexisting liver disease) are critically ill. All surgery other than liver transplantation is contraindicated in these patients.

Operative Risk Assessment

Chronic hepatitis

Chronic hepatitis is characterized by persistent liver inflammation for greater than 6 months duration. A variety of viral, genetic, autoimmune, metabolic, and drug-induced causes of chronic hepatitis have been identified. Regardless of the cause, the histopathologic findings are classified by the grade of necroinflammatory activity and stage of fibrosis. If a patient is found preoperatively to have chronic hepatitis, treatment of the underlying disease can often reduce necroinflammatory activity and may even reverse fibrosis.

Surgical risk in patients with chronic hepatitis and without cirrhosis correlates with the clinical, biochemical, and histologic severity of the disease. A patient's perioperative risk may be linked to the grade of inflammation, although little is known about the predictive value of hepatic inflammation alone. The few published studies of the risk of surgery in patients with mild to moderate chronic hepatitis without cirrhosis suggest that such patients are at no additional surgical risk.[17,18] Patients with biochemically and histologically severe chronic hepatitis have an increased surgical risk, particularly when hepatic synthetic or excretory function is impaired, portal hypertension is present, or bridging or multilobular necrosis are found on a liver biopsy specimen.

Cirrhosis

Cirrhosis is characterized by parenchymal necrosis, fibrosis, nodular regeneration, and vasculature distortion leading to portal hypertension. Decompensated cirrhosis is defined as the presence of ascites, hepatic encephalopathy, varices, hepatorenal syndrome, or synthetic dysfunction (such as hypoalbuminemia or prolongation of the prothrombin time). Surgical risk is increased in patients with cirrhosis. The magnitude of perioperative risk correlates with the degree of hepatic decompensation.

Stratification by Child class Although the optimal measure of hepatic decompensation in patients with cirrhosis remains unclear, since the 1970s the standard for assessing perioperative morbidity and mortality in patients with cirrhosis has been the CTP scoring system based on the patient's serum bilirubin and albumin levels, prothrombin time, and severity of encephalopathy and ascites.[1] The studies that led to this standard have all been retrospective and limited to a small number of highly selected patients, but the results have been remarkably consistent. Two of the most important studies, separated by 13 years, reported nearly identical results: mortality rates for patients undergoing surgery were 10% for those with Child class A, 30% for those with Child class B, and 76% to 82% for those with Child class C cirrhosis (**Table 1**).[19,20] In addition to predicting perioperative mortality, the Child class correlates with the frequency of postoperative complications, which include liver failure, worsening encephalopathy, bleeding, infection, renal failure, hypoxia, and intractable ascites.

Even in patients with Child class A cirrhosis, the risk of perioperative morbidity is increased when there is associated portal hypertension. Postoperative morbidity in such patients may be reduced by preoperative placement of a transjugular intrahepatic portosystemic shunt (TIPSS).[21,22]

Several factors other than the Child class can increase the perioperative risk. Emergency surgery is associated with a higher mortality rate than elective surgery: 22% versus 10% for patients in Child class A; 38% versus 30% for those in Child class B; and 100% versus 82% for those in Child class C.[20] A diagnosis of chronic obstructive lung disease and surgery on the respiratory tract are also independent risk factors for perioperative mortality in patients with cirrhosis.[23]

The general consensus is that elective surgery is well tolerated in patients with Child class A cirrhosis, permissible with preoperative preparation in patients with Child class B cirrhosis (except those undergoing extensive hepatic resection or cardiac surgery, see later discussion), and contraindicated in patients with Child class C cirrhosis.[24]

Stratification by MELD score The MELD score was created to predict mortality after TIPSS, then extended to risk stratify patients awaiting liver transplantation, and more recently to predict perioperative mortality.[25] The MELD score is a linear regression model based on serum bilirubin, creatinine levels, and international normalized ratio (INR). It has several distinct advantages over the Child classification: it is objective, weights the variables, and does not rely on arbitrary cutoff values. One study showed that each 1 point increase in the MELD score makes an incremental contribution to risk, thereby suggesting that the MELD score increases precision in predicting postoperative mortality.[26]

Several studies have examined the MELD score as a predictor of surgical mortality in patients with cirrhosis (see **Table 1**). In a retrospective study of 140 patients with cirrhosis who underwent surgery, a 1% increase in mortality for each 1 point increase in the MELD score from 5 to 20 and a 2% increase in mortality for each 1 point increase in the MELD score greater than 20 was seen.[27] The largest retrospective study of the MELD score as a predictor of perioperative mortality, by Teh and colleagues,[28] evaluated 772 patients with cirrhosis who underwent abdominal (other than laparoscopic cholecystectomy), orthopedic, and cardiovascular surgery. The patients' median preoperative MELD score was 8, and few had a MELD score greater than 15. In addition, most patients had a platelet count greater than 60,000/μL and an INR less than 1.5. In this selected cohort, patients with a MELD score of 7 or less had a mortality

Table 1
Mortality rates associated with specific types of surgery in patients with cirrhosis

Type of Surgery and References	Number of Patients in Study(ies)	Overall	Mortality, %				MELD Score
			Child Class				
			A	B	C		
Appendectomy[88]	69	9	NA	NA	NA		NA
Cardiac[58,59]	44, 18	16–17	0–3	42–50	100		NA
Cholecystectomy[45,48]	226, 33	1–3	0.5	3	NA		<8 = 0% ≥8 = 6%
Colorectal cancer surgery[89]	72	12.5	6	13	27		NA
Esophagectomy[90]	18	17	NA	NA	NA		NA
Hepatic resection[66–68]	587, 154, 82	9	9[a]	NA	NA		<9 = 0% ≥9 = 29%
Major abdominal surgery[19,20]	100, 92	26–30	10	30–31	76–82		NA
Total knee arthroplasty[91]	51	0	0	NA	NA		NA
Treatment of hepatic hydrothorax with talc[92]	18	39	NA	NA	NA		NA

Abbreviation: NA, not available.
[a] The exact number of Child class B patients was not available for the largest study; however, almost all patients had Child class A cirrhosis.

rate of 5.7%; patients with a MELD score of 8 to 11 had a mortality rate of 10.3%; and patients with a MELD score of 12 to 15 had a mortality rate of 25.4% (**Fig. 1**). The increase in relative risk of death was almost linear for MELD scores greater than 8.

In addition to the MELD score, the American Society of Anesthesiologists (ASA) class (**Table 2**) and the patient's age were shown by Teh and colleagues[28] to contribute to postoperative mortality risk. An ASA class of IV added the equivalent of 5.5 MELD points to the mortality rate, whereas an ASA class of V was associated with a 100% mortality rate. The influence of the ASA class was greatest in the first 7 days after surgery, after which the MELD score became the principal determinant of risk. In this study,[28] no patient younger than 30 years died, and an age older than 70 years added the equivalent of 3 MELD points to the mortality rate. Unlike studies that evaluated the ability of the Child class to predict surgical mortality, emergency surgery was not an independent predictor of mortality when the MELD score was used, because patients who underwent emergency surgery had higher MELD scores.

Based on the study of Teh and colleagues,[28] a Web site (http://www.mayoclinic.org/meld/mayomodel9.html) can be used to calculate 7-day, 30-day, 90-day, 1-year, and 5-year surgical mortality risk based on a patient's age, ASA class, INR, and serum bilirubin and creatinine levels (the last 3 items constitute the MELD score). Use of the MELD score and Child class are not mutually exclusive and may complement one another, but the MELD score is probably the most precise single predictor of perioperative mortality.

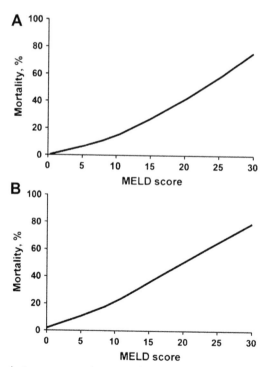

Fig. 1. Relationship between operative mortality and MELD score in 772 patients with cirrhosis who underwent surgery in 1980 to 1990 and 1994 to 2004. (*A*) Thirty-day mortality; (*B*) 90-day mortality. For patients with a MELD score greater than 8, each 1 point increase in the MELD score was associated with a 14% increase in both 30-day and 90-day mortality rates. (*From* Teh SH, Nagorney DM, Stevens SR, et al. Risk factors for mortality after surgery in patients with cirrhosis. Gastroenterology 2007;132(4):1261–9; with permission.)

Table 2	
American Society of Anesthesiologists (ASA) classification	
Class	
I	Healthy patient
II	Patient with mild systemic disease without functional limitation
III	Patient with severe systemic disease with functional limitation
IV	Patient with severe systemic disease that is a constant threat to life
V	Moribund patient not expected to survive >24 h with or without surgery
E	Emergent nature of surgery (added to classification I–V above)

Specific causes of liver disease

Chronic hepatitis B and C More than 350 million people worldwide and 1.25 million people in the United States are chronically infected with hepatitis B virus (HBV).[29,30] Inactive carriers of HBV, who have normal serum aminotransferase levels and no hepatic inflammation, are not at increased risk for postoperative complications, but patients with chronic hepatitis B, with or without cirrhosis, may be at increased risk of operative morbidity if they have significant hepatic inflammation or dysfunction. In patients treated with nucleoside or nucleotide analogues, therapy for chronic HBV should not be interrupted in the perioperative period; hepatitis flares can occur following cessation of therapy, and interruption of treatment may allow viral resistance to develop.

An estimated 170 million people worldwide and 1.6% of the United States population are chronically infected with hepatitis C virus (HCV).[31,32] Patients with chronic HCV infection typically have elevated serum aminotransferase levels ranging from 1.3 to 3 times the upper limit of normal, although levels may be within normal limits. The impact of the presence of antibodies to HCV on surgical outcome has been studied retrospectively in United States veterans, and in the absence of cirrhosis, HCV infection does not increase the morbidity or mortality of surgery.[18] Patients undergoing therapy for HCV infection may experience myelosuppression due to peginterferon and hemolytic anemia due to ribavirin; leukopenia, when present, may contribute to functional immunosuppression. Treatment-induced thrombocytopenia, if severe, may contribute to operative bleeding. In general, however, peginterferon and ribavirin therapy should not be discontinued without consulting the patient's treating physician.

Nonalcoholic fatty liver disease Nonalcoholic fatty liver disease (NAFLD) encompasses a spectrum from bland steatosis, to nonalcoholic steatohepatitis (NASH), to cirrhosis. Given the current epidemic of obesity, an increasing number of patients with NAFLD are undergoing surgery. More than 90% of morbidly obese patients who undergo bariatric surgery have histologic evidence of hepatic steatosis, and up to 6% are found intraoperatively to have cirrhosis.[33,34] Patients with NAFLD but without cirrhosis do not seem to have increased mortality following elective surgery. Patients with compensated cirrhosis caused by NASH may be considered candidates for bariatric surgery, because weight loss improves hepatic inflammation and in some cases fibrosis.[35–37] Even though patients with NAFLD do not have an increased risk of perioperative mortality from their liver disease, this population is at higher risk for diabetes, hypertension, hypertriglyceridemia, and coronary heart disease.[38,39] As a result, preoperative cardiac risk stratification is essential.

A trend toward increased mortality following hepatic resection has been observed in patients with moderate to severe hepatic steatosis (greater than 30% of hepatocytes containing fat) despite the absence of cirrhosis, probably because steatosis inhibits hepatic regeneration.[40]

Other causes Surgery in patients with Wilson disease can precipitate or aggravate neuropsychiatric symptoms. Treatment with D-penicillamine, a copper chelator, interferes with the cross-linking of collagen and may impair wound healing.[41] As a result, the dose of D-penicillamine should be decreased before planned surgery and during the first several postoperative weeks.

Patients with hemochromatosis should be evaluated preoperatively for additional complications of iron overload, especially diabetes and cardiomyopathy. Although original reports suggested lower survival rates for liver transplantation in patients with hemochromatosis, compared with patients who had other causes of cirrhosis, subsequent reports have noted survival outcomes similar to those for other indications.[42]

Autoimmune hepatitis in remission is not a contraindication to elective surgery in patients with compensated hepatic function. Patients receiving chronic glucocorticoid therapy should be given appropriate stress doses during the perioperative period.

Patients with α-1 antitrypsin deficiency are at risk for liver and lung disease. Therefore, careful evaluation of the patient's pulmonary status should be undertaken before surgery, and pulmonary function testing should be performed when pulmonary dysfunction is suspected.

OPERATIVE RISK ASSOCIATED WITH SPECIFIC TYPES OF SURGERY
Biliary Tract Surgery

Biliary tract surgery of any kind, including cholecystectomy, presents unique challenges in patients with cirrhosis because of the combination of portal hypertension and coagulopathy. An increased risk of bleeding should be anticipated in patients with advanced cirrhosis as demonstrated by a prolonged prothrombin time or thrombocytopenia, although the actual risk of bleeding does not correlate with the degree of coagulopathy.[43,44]

Patients with cirrhosis are at increased risk of gallstone formation and associated complications when compared with noncirrhotic persons. In a case–control study of patients who underwent cholecystectomy, a MELD score of 8 or more had a sensitivity of 91% and specificity of 77% for predicting 90-day postoperative morbidity.[45] In general, laparoscopic cholecystectomy is permissible for patients with Child class A cirrhosis and selected patients with Child class B cirrhosis without portal hypertension.[46–48] In contrast, in patients with Child class C cirrhosis, cholecystostomy, rather than cholecystectomy, is recommended; however, when surgery is deemed the only option, an open rather than laparoscopic approach is recommended.

In addition to jaundice reflecting hepatocellular dysfunction, cirrhotic patients can present with jaundice due to biliary obstruction. In a patient with a benign cause for obstructive jaundice or a malignant cause not amenable to curative surgery, nonsurgical approaches to decompression using endoscopic retrograde cholangiopancreatography (ERCP) or percutaneous transhepatic cholangiography should be explored. Before ERCP was widely used, a study of patients with obstructive jaundice indentified 3 key predictors of mortality: a hematocrit value less than 30%, an initial serum bilirubin level greater than 11 mg/dL (200 μmol/L), and a malignant cause of obstruction.[49] When all 3 factors were present, the mortality rate approached 60%; when none was present, it was only 5%. Not surprisingly, malignant biliary obstruction carried a dramatically higher operative mortality rate (26.1%) than benign biliary obstruction (3.7%). In addition, patients with obstructive jaundice are at increased risk of bacterial infections, disseminated intravascular coagulation, gastrointestinal bleeding, delayed wound healing, wound dehiscence, incisional hernias, and renal failure. Routine preoperative decompression of an obstructed biliary tree does not seem to reduce subsequent operative mortality.

Intestinal barrier integrity may be compromised in patients with obstructive jaundice and cirrhosis, leading to increased permeability to microorganisms.[50,51] Furthermore, patients with cirrhosis are immunosuppressed due to reticuloendothelial cell and neutrophil dysfunction.[52] Bacterial translocation because of Kupffer cell dysfunction can lead to bacteremia and endotoxemia. The paucity of bile salts in the gastrointestinal tract resulting in obstructive jaundice enhances intestinal absorption of endotoxin. Limited evidence suggests that administration of lactulose to patients with obstructive jaundice may prevent endotoxemia,[53,54] but it is not clear that any additional clinical benefit occurs when lactulose is added to the administration of antibiotics and careful attention is paid to the patient's intraoperative hemodynamic and volume status.[55]

Endoscopic or percutaneous biliary drainage is preferable to surgery for benign conditions in cirrhotic patients. Although endoscopic sphincterotomy is associated with an increased risk of bleeding in these patients, morbidity and mortality rates are low even in patients with Child class C cirrhosis.[56] In patients with coagulopathy or thrombocytopenia, endoscopic papillary balloon dilation is associated with a lower risk of bleeding than standard sphincterotomy and is preferred despite a possibly higher risk of pancreatitis.[57]

Cardiac Surgery

Cardiac surgery and other procedures requiring cardiopulmonary bypass are associated with greater mortality in patients with cirrhosis than are most other surgical procedures. Risk factors for hepatic decompensation following cardiac surgery include the total time on bypass, use of pulsatile as opposed to nonpulsatile bypass flow, and need for perioperative vasopressor support. Cardiopulmonary bypass can exacerbate underlying coagulopathy by inducing platelet dysfunction, fibrinolysis, and hypocalcemia.

In 2 retrospective series of patients who underwent surgery requiring cardiopulmonary bypass, low mortality rates were observed in those with Child class A cirrhosis (0% [0/10] and 3% [1/31]) but rates were markedly increased in those with Child class B (42%–50%) and C (100%, n = 2) cirrhosis. In addition, more than 75% of Child class B and C patients experienced hepatic decompensation.[58,59] Increased mortality is also predicted by an increased MELD score. A MELD score greater than 13 predicted a poor prognosis, although no safe cutoff score could be established. Therefore, a CTP score of 7 or less (Child class A) or a low MELD score suggests that cardiopulmonary bypass can be accomplished safely in patients with cirrhosis.

In addition to an elevated CTP or MELD score, clinically significant portal hypertension is a contraindication to cardiothoracic surgery. Portal decompression with TIPS placement may make the risk acceptable if the CTP and MELD scores remain low[60]; however, elevated right-sided cardiac pressures from cardiac dysfunction and pulmonary hypertension are absolute contraindications to TIPSS placement.

In general, the least invasive option—angioplasty with or without stent placement—should be considered whenever feasible in a patient with advanced cirrhosis who requires coronary artery revascularization. The type of stent used is important as coated stents require longer use of aspirin and clopidogrel than do uncoated stents. In addition, the patient's likelihood of requiring surgery after coronary artery intervention and risk of bleeding due to coagulopathy or thrombocytopenia should be taken into consideration.

Hepatic Resection

Hepatocellular carcinoma (HCC) occurs in patients with cirrhosis at a rate of approximately 1% to 4% per year.[61–63] As a result, screening of patients with cirrhosis is recommended,[64] and many HCCs are now detected that may be amenable to resection. Patients with cirrhosis who undergo hepatic resection for HCC or other benign or malignant tumors are at increased risk of hepatic decompensation and mortality compared with cirrhotic patients who undergo other types of surgery. These patients lose functional hepatocellular mass in the setting of an already compromised hepatic reserve. In addition, underlying NAFLD, if present, inhibits hepatic regeneration postoperatively, further increasing the risk of hepatic decompensation.[40]

Mortality rates as high as 25% are reported following hepatic resection in patients with cirrhosis.[65] Risk stratification based on the Child class and MELD score have allowed more appropriate selection of patients, thus leading to lower mortality rates. In an analysis of 82 cirrhotic patients who underwent hepatic resection, the perioperative mortality rate was 29% in patients with a MELD score of 9 or more but 0% in those with a MELD score of 8 or less.[66] Another study identified Child class and ASA class, but not MELD score, as significant predictors of outcome following liver resection. In this study, the mean MELD score was low (6.5), which likely limited the ability of the MELD score to discriminate between risk groups.[67]

In addition to predicting mortality, the MELD score can predict morbidity after liver resection. In one study,[68] the frequency of liver failure post-resection was 0%, 3.6%, and 37.5% in patients with MELD scores of less than 9, 9 to 10, and greater than 10, respectively.

The effect of chronic viral hepatitis on surgical outcome in patients with cirrhosis and compensated hepatic function is uncertain. In a series of 172 patients with HCV-related HCC who underwent hepatic resection, the outcome was best predicted by tumor-related factors, including the serum α-fetoprotein level and tumor vascular invasion.[69] In contrast, another study suggested that the risk of recurrent HCC may be higher and overall long-term survival poorer following hepatectomy for patients with HCC and chronic viral hepatitis compared with patients who have HCC without viral hepatitis.[70]

Despite better outcomes in recent years, likely resulting from better patient selection, 5-year HCC recurrence rates are as high as 100%, and 5-year survival rates are no higher than 55%.[24,71,72] The high recurrence and mortality rates reflect the underlying liver disease, which leads either to the development of a new or recurrent liver cancer or worsening hepatic synthetic dysfunction. As a result, liver transplantation is often advised in acceptable candidates, even in patients with Child class A cirrhosis, in regions where timely transplantation can be accomplished.[71–73]

Nonsurgical options for treating HCC include radiofrequency ablation, microwave ablation, ethanol injection, transarterial chemoembolization, and intrahepatic yttrium-90 microsphere radioembolization. These options are currently applied in patients awaiting liver transplantation and in those who are not surgical candidates.[73] Although only surgical options are considered potentially curative, combinations of nonsurgical methods have improved long-term survival over single-modality therapy.[74]

Endoscopic Procedures

Patients with cirrhosis should be screened for esophageal varices by upper gastrointestinal endoscopy. Moderate (conscious) sedation does not increase mortality in patients with cirrhosis who do not have clinically overt hepatic encephalopathy. Coagulopathy and thrombocytopenia do not increase the risk associated with variceal band ligation but may influence the approach to endoscopic tissue acquisition and the treatment of bleeding from lesions other than varices.

Gastrostomy tube placement generally should be avoided in patients with cirrhosis and is contraindicated in patients with ascites, because of a high risk of leakage and infection. In addition, enlarged intraabdominal veins may be inadvertently punctured during blind percutaneous trocar placement in patients with portal hypertension.

PERIOPERATIVE CARE
Coagulopathy

In patients with liver disease, impaired hemostasis reflects decreased production of clotting factors because of hepatic synthetic dysfunction and, in some cirrhotics, depletion of vitamin K stores due to malnutrition or decreased intestinal absorption. Increased fibrinolytic activity with laboratory features of mild disseminated intravascular coagulation are also frequent in patients with cirrhosis. Thrombocytopenia due to portal hypertension-induced splenic sequestration and alcohol-induced bone marrow suppression is common.

Subcutaneous administration of vitamin K, 10 mg/d for 1 to 3 days, will correct coagulopathy due to nutritional or bile salt deficiency but not due to hepatic synthetic dysfunction. Transfusion of fresh frozen plasma and platelets may be necessary perioperatively in patients with marked coagulopathy or thrombocytopenia, respectively, to permit safe surgery. The risk of surgery in patients with severe coagulopathy and thrombocytopenia (defined as an INR >1.5 and platelets <50,000/mm^3, respectively) has not been studied and is uncertain. Cryoprecipitate, which contains large quantities of von Willebrand multimers and is rich in fibrinogen, should be considered when hemorrhage cannot be controlled. A prolonged bleeding time also can be treated with diamino-8-D-arginine vasopressin.

Recombinant factor VIIa has been introduced as an additional option for the treatment of bleeding due to coagulopathy in cirrhotic patients undergoing surgery. In a randomized, controlled trial of cirrhotic patients undergoing liver transplantation, patients randomized to perioperative recombinant factor VIIa were less likely to require packed red blood cell transfusions than patients randomized to placebo.[75] Because of the high cost, transient effect, absence of data showing improved outcomes, and theoretical concern about an increased risk of thromboembolic events, recombinant factor VIIa should only be used when bleeding cannot be controlled by other means. Optimal surgical technique and maintenance of a low central venous pressure may reduce blood loss.[76]

Ascites

Ascites with or without hepatic hydrothorax can compromise respiration. Following abdominal surgery, ascites increases the risk of wound dehiscence and abdominal wall herniation. Although ascites can be drained at the time of abdominal surgery, it typically reaccumulates within days. Therefore, preoperative control of ascites with diuretics or TIPS placement is advisable. Medical therapy for ascites includes salt restriction to 2 g/d with the combination of spironolactone and furosemide, beginning at daily doses of 100 mg and 40 mg, respectively.

An umbilical hernia is a frequent complication of ascites and can be at risk of incarceration or spontaneous rupture. Elective surgical umbilical hernia repair, either with or without mesh prosthesis, may be considered only in carefully selected patients with decompensated cirrhosis.[77] TIPSS placement should be considered in patients with difficult to control ascites and those with rupture of an umbilical hernia.[78]

Renal Dysfunction

Renal dysfunction is a dreaded complication in patients with cirrhosis. Advanced liver disease is associated with increased levels of endogenous vasodilators, which lead to peripheral vasodilatation, a chronic hyperdynamic circulation, and low blood pressure. Among the clinical consequences of a hyperdynamic circulation is activation of the sympathetic nervous system and renin–angiotensin–aldosterone axis. Elevated levels of renal vasodilatory prostaglandins attempt to compensate for the vasoconstrictive influence of angiotensin, and when this fails, hepatorenal syndrome develops. The impact of hepatorenal syndrome on mortality is well established and accounts for inclusion of the serum creatinine level in the MELD score. In patients with cirrhosis, however, the serum creatinine level often overestimates the actual glomerular filtration rate because of muscle wasting and decreased urea synthesis.

Perioperative renal dysfunction in a patient with cirrhosis may be the result of intravascular volume depletion, nephrotoxicity, acute tubular necrosis, or hepatorenal syndrome. It is imperative to differentiate among these possibilities. Cirrhotic patients may be intravascularly volume depleted but total body volume overloaded, and this possibility should always be considered first in patients with cirrhosis in whom renal dysfunction develops. Diuretics and a fluid challenge should be initiated, and potential nephrotoxins (aminoglycoside antibiotics, nonsteroidal anti-inflammatory agents, intravenous contrast agents) should be discontinued or avoided.

In an attempt to avoid acute tubular necrosis and hepatorenal syndrome perioperatively, the patient's volume status, urine output, and systemic perfusion should be monitored assiduously. Intravenous infusions of salt-poor albumin or blood are widely used in lieu of crystalloid fluid replacement in patients with liver disease, despite a lack of data supporting an advantage to this approach.

Treatment of hepatorenal syndrome can be attempted with the combination of the oral α-agonist midodrine, subcutaneous octreotide, and intravenous salt-poor albumin.[79] Another strategy includes intravenous norepinephrine (titrated to increase mean arterial blood pressure by 10 mm Hg) plus intravenous salt-poor albumin.[80] In patients who fail to respond to medical therapy, TIPSS can be attempted if the MELD score remains low.[81]

Hepatorenal syndrome is a terminal event unless patients are treated successfully or transplanted. Therefore, surgery other than liver transplantation is unlikely to change a patient's prognosis in this setting.

Encephalopathy

Hepatic encephalopathy is a state of disordered central nervous system function characterized by disturbances in consciousness, behavior, and personality.[82] The diagnosis of hepatic encephalopathy should be made clinically by evaluating the patient for personality changes, sleep disturbances, tremor, hyperreflexia, and asterixis. Later stages of encephalopathy are associated with frank confusion, stupor, and coma. An elevated serum arterial or venous ammonia level is present in patients with encephalopathy but is not specific. The serum ammonia level may be useful, however, in patients in whom the diagnosis of encephalopathy is unclear, such as those with concomitant psychiatric or neurologic disorders or sedated patients.

Elective surgery should be deferred until hepatic encephalopathy has been controlled, because precipitating factors are inevitable in the postoperative period. Precipitants include volume contraction, hypokalemia, infection, bleeding, and use of sedative or psychoactive medications. Even for patients without overt hepatic decompensation, some degree of encephalopathy may be encountered following surgery. Despite the high frequency of subclinical encephalopathy in patients with cirrhosis, no compelling data support a role for prophylactic therapy to prevent encephalopathy in patients undergoing surgery. Risk factors should be minimized by ensuring adequate volume resuscitation, repleting potassium, controlling infection and bleeding, and minimizing the use of narcotics and other sedating medications.

Oral or rectal (as retention enemas) lactulose is often used to treat hepatic encephalopathy. Lactulose should be titrated to 2 to 3 soft stools daily, and electrolyte abnormalities and volume depletion should be avoided. Oral antibiotics such as rifaximin, neomycin, or metronidazole may also be used, and rifaximin is increasingly preferred as a first-line antibiotic agent.[83]

Gastroesophageal Varices

Whether surgery per se is a risk factor for variceal bleeding is uncertain. For patients with known large varices, elective cardiothoracic and probably major abdominal surgery should only be considered after TIPSS placement. For patients with known varices who undergo minor surgery, primary prophylaxis with either a nonselective oral β-adrenergic antagonist (eg, propranolol, nadolol) or endoscopic band ligation should be instituted.[84] Patients with prior variceal bleeding who undergo minor surgery should be treated, if necessary, with band ligation and β-blockade or TIPSS placement.

Nutrition

All patients with chronic liver disease are at high risk for protein-energy malnutrition. Patients with cholestatic liver disease are also at risk for fat-soluble vitamin malabsorption. Persons with alcohol-induced liver disease are often deficient in thiamine and folate and have depleted levels of total body potassium and magnesium. Nutritional deficiencies among these patients are often underdiagnosed. Clinical clues to nutritional deficiencies include muscle wasting, ascites, and hypoalbuminemia, which may not be solely attributable to hepatic synthetic dysfunction.[85]

Poor nutritional status impacts the prognosis adversely in patients with cirrhosis in general.[86] In addition, mortality is increased after general surgical procedures or liver transplantation in malnourished patients.[87] Whenever possible, a patient's nutritional status should be addressed before elective surgery. Enteral nutritional supplementation seems to improve immunocompetence and short-term prognosis in patients with cirrhosis and is the preferred approach. Percutaneous gastrostomy, as discussed earlier, is contraindicated in patients with ascites or suspected abdominal wall varices. Central venous catheterization for parenteral nutrition carries a risk of infectious and bleeding complications and should be avoided whenever possible.

Postoperative Monitoring

Postoperatively, patients with cirrhosis need to be monitored for the development of signs of hepatic decompensation, including encephalopathy, coagulopathy, ascites, worsening jaundice, and renal dysfunction. If any of these indicators are found, supportive therapy should be initiated immediately. The prothrombin time is the single best indicator of hepatic synthetic function. An elevated serum bilirubin level can indicate worsening hepatic function but can occur for other reasons, including blood transfusion, resorption of extravasated blood, or infection. Renal function must be monitored closely. If renal dysfunction is found, the course should be pursued aggressively and treatment initiated.

Hypoglycemia may occur in patients with decompensated cirrhosis or acute liver failure as a result of depleted hepatic glycogen stores and impaired gluconeogenesis.

Serum glucose levels should be monitored closely if postoperative liver failure is suspected.

Careful attention should be paid to the assessment of intravascular volume, which is often difficult to assess in the setting of extravascular volume overload. Intravascular volume maintenance minimizes the risk of hepatic and renal underperfusion. On the other hand, infusion of too much crystalloid may lead to acute hepatic congestion, increased venous oozing, and pulmonary edema and to postoperative ascites, peripheral edema, and wound dehiscence.

SUMMARY

Surgery is performed more frequently now than in the past in patients with cirrhosis, in part because of the long-term survival of patients with advanced liver disease. Estimation of perioperative mortality is limited by the retrospective nature of and biased patient selection in the available clinical studies. Use of the Child classification and MELD score provides a reasonably precise estimation of perioperative mortality but does not replace the need for careful preoperative preparation and postoperative monitoring, as early detection of complications is essential to improve outcomes.

REFERENCES

1. Friedman LS. The risk of surgery in patients with liver disease. Hepatology 1999; 29(6):1617–23.
2. Gholson CF, Provenza JM, Bacon BR. Hepatologic considerations in patients with parenchymal liver disease undergoing surgery. Am J Gastroenterol 1990;85(5): 487–96.
3. Gelman S. General anesthesia and hepatic circulation. Can J Physiol Pharmacol 1987;65(8):1762–79.
4. Sato K, Kawamura T, Wakusawa R. Hepatic blood flow and function in elderly patients undergoing laparoscopic cholecystectomy. Anesth Analg 2000;90(5): 1198–202.
5. Rodriguez-Roisin R, Krowka MJ. Hepatopulmonary syndrome—a liver-induced lung vascular disorder. N Engl J Med 2008;358(22):2378–87.
6. Kawut SM, Krowka MJ, Trotter JF, et al. Clinical risk factors for portopulmonary hypertension. Hepatology 2008;48(1):196–203.
7. Lai HC, Wang KY, Lee WL, et al. Severe pulmonary hypertension complicates postoperative outcome of non-cardiac surgery. Br J Anaesth 2007;99(2):184–90.
8. Kharasch ED, Hankins D, Mautz D, et al. Identification of the enzyme responsible for oxidative halothane metabolism: implications for prevention of halothane hepatitis. Lancet 1996;347(9012):1367–71.
9. Nishiyama T, Fujimoto T, Hanaoka K. A comparison of liver function after hepatectomy in cirrhotic patients between sevoflurane and isoflurane in anesthesia with nitrous oxide and epidural block. Anesth Analg 2004;98(4):990–3.
10. Servin F, Desmonts JM, Haberer JP, et al. Pharmacokinetics and protein binding of propofol in patients with cirrhosis. Anesthesiology 1988;69(6):887–91.
11. Ioannou GN, Boyko EJ, Lee SP. The prevalence and predictors of elevated serum aminotransferase activity in the United States in 1999–2002. Am J Gastroenterol 2006;101(1):76–82.
12. Ioannou GN, Weiss NS, Boyko EJ, et al. Elevated serum alanine aminotransferase activity and calculated risk of coronary heart disease in the United States. Hepatology 2006;43(5):1145–51.

13. Strauss AA, Siegfried SF, Schwartz AH, et al. Liver decompression by drainage of the common bile duct in subacute and chronic jaundice: report of seventy-three cases with hepatitis or concomitant biliary duct infection as cause. Am J Surg 1958;97:137–40.

14. Harville DD, Summerskill WH. Surgery in acute hepatitis. Causes and effects. JAMA 1963;184:257–61.

15. Ceccanti M, Attili A, Balducci G, et al. Acute alcoholic hepatitis. J Clin Gastroenterol 2006;40(9):833–41.

16. Greenwood SM, Leffler CT, Minkowitz S. The increased mortality rate of open liver biopsy in alcoholic hepatitis. Surg Gynecol Obstet 1972;134(4):600–4.

17. Runyon BA. Surgical procedures are well tolerated by patients with asymptomatic chronic hepatitis. J Clin Gastroenterol 1986;8(5):542–4.

18. Cheung RC, Hsieh F, Wang Y, et al. The impact of hepatitis C status on postoperative outcome. Anesth Analg 2003;97(2):550–4.

19. Garrison RN, Cryer HM, Howard DA, et al. Clarification of risk factors for abdominal operations in patients with hepatic cirrhosis. Ann Surg 1984;199(6): 648–55.

20. Mansour A, Watson W, Shayani V, et al. Abdominal operations in patients with cirrhosis: still a major surgical challenge. Surgery 1997;122(4):730–5.

21. Gil A, Martinez-Regueira F, Hernandez-Lizoain JL, et al. The role of transjugular intrahepatic portosystemic shunt prior to abdominal tumoral surgery in cirrhotic patients with portal hypertension. Eur J Surg Oncol 2004;30(1):46–52.

22. Azoulay D, Buabse F, Damiano I, et al. Neoadjuvant transjugular intrahepatic portosystemic shunt: a solution for extrahepatic abdominal operation in cirrhotic patients with severe portal hypertension. J Am Coll Surg 2001;193(1):46–51.

23. Ziser A, Plevak DJ, Wiesner RH, et al. Morbidity and mortality in cirrhotic patients undergoing anesthesia and surgery. Anesthesiology 1999;90(1):42–53.

24. MacIntosh EL, Minuk GY. Hepatic resection in patients with cirrhosis and hepatocellular carcinoma. Surg Gynecol Obstet 1992;174(3):245–54.

25. Malinchoc M, Kamath PS, Gordon FD, et al. A model to predict poor survival in patients undergoing transjugular intrahepatic portosystemic shunts. Hepatology 2000;31(4):864–71.

26. O'Leary JG, Friedman LS. Predicting surgical risk in patients with cirrhosis: from art to science. Gastroenterology 2007;132(4):1609–11.

27. Northup PG, Wanamaker RC, Lee VD, et al. Model for End-Stage Liver Disease (MELD) predicts nontransplant surgical mortality in patients with cirrhosis. Ann Surg 2005;242(2):244–51.

28. Teh SH, Nagorney DM, Stevens SR, et al. Risk factors for mortality after surgery in patients with cirrhosis. Gastroenterology 2007;132(4):1261–9.

29. Lavanchy D. Hepatitis B virus epidemiology, disease burden, treatment, and current and emerging prevention and control measures. J Viral Hepat 2004;11(2):97–107.

30. McQuillan GM, Coleman PJ, Kruszon-Moran D, et al. Prevalence of hepatitis B virus infection in the United States: the National Health and Nutrition Examination Surveys, 1976 through 1994. Am J Public Health 1999;89(1):14–8.

31. Armstrong GL, Wasley A, Simard EP, et al. The prevalence of hepatitis C virus infection in the United States, 1999 through 2002. Ann Intern Med 2006;144(10):705–14.

32. Global surveillance and control of hepatitis C. Report of a WHO Consultation organized in collaboration with the Viral Hepatitis Prevention Board, Antwerp, Belgium. J Viral Hepat 1999;6(1):35–47.

33. Brolin RE, Bradley LJ, Taliwal RV. Unsuspected cirrhosis discovered during elective obesity operations. Arch Surg 1998;133(1):84–8.

34. Machado M, Marques-Vidal P, Cortez-Pinto H. Hepatic histology in obese patients undergoing bariatric surgery. J Hepatol 2006;45(4):600–6.
35. Barker KB, Palekar NA, Bowers SP, et al. Non-alcoholic steatohepatitis: effect of Roux-en-Y gastric bypass surgery. Am J Gastroenterol 2006;101(2):368–73.
36. Furuya CK, de Oliveira CP, de Mello ES, et al. Effects of bariatric surgery on nonalcoholic fatty liver disease: preliminary findings after 2 years. J Gastroenterol Hepatol 2007;22(4):510–4.
37. Liu X, Lazenby AJ, Clements RH, et al. Resolution of nonalcoholic steatohepatits after gastric bypass surgery. Obes Surg 2007;17(4):486–92.
38. Hamaguchi M, Kojima T, Takeda N, et al. Nonalcoholic fatty liver disease is a novel predictor of cardiovascular disease. World J Gastroenterol 2007;13(10):1579–84.
39. Targher G, Arcaro G. Non-alcoholic fatty liver disease and increased risk of cardiovascular disease. Atherosclerosis 2007;191(2):235–40.
40. Selzner M, Clavien PA. Fatty liver in liver transplantation and surgery. Semin Liver Dis 2001;21(1):105–13.
41. Roberts EA, Schilsky ML. Diagnosis and treatment of Wilson disease: an update. Hepatology 2008;47(6):2089–111.
42. Yu L, Ioannou GN. Survival of liver transplant recipients with hemochromatosis in the United States. Gastroenterology 2007;133(2):489–95.
43. Schiff J, Misra M, Rendon G, et al. Laparoscopic cholecystectomy in cirrhotic patients. Surg Endosc 2005;19(9):1278–81.
44. Tripodi A, Caldwell SH, Hoffman M, et al. Review article: the prothrombin time test as a measure of bleeding risk and prognosis in liver disease. Aliment Pharmacol Ther 2007;26(2):141–8.
45. Perkins L, Jeffries M, Patel T. Utility of preoperative scores for predicting morbidity after cholecystectomy in patients with cirrhosis. Clin Gastroenterol Hepatol 2004;2(12):1123–8.
46. Curro G, Baccarani U, Adani G, et al. Laparoscopic cholecystectomy in patients with mild cirrhosis and symptomatic cholelithiasis. Transplant Proc 2007;39(5):1471–3.
47. Poggio JL, Rowland CM, Gores GJ, et al. A comparison of laparoscopic and open cholecystectomy in patients with compensated cirrhosis and symptomatic gallstone disease. Surgery 2000;127(4):405–11.
48. Yeh CN, Chen MF, Jan YY. Laparoscopic cholecystectomy in 226 cirrhotic patients. Experience of a single center in Taiwan. Surg Endosc 2002;16(11):1583–7.
49. Dixon JM, Armstrong CP, Duffy SW, et al. Factors affecting morbidity and mortality after surgery for obstructive jaundice: a review of 373 patients. Gut 1983;24(9):845–52.
50. Keshavarzian A, Holmes EW, Patel M, et al. Leaky gut in alcoholic cirrhosis: a possible mechanism for alcohol-induced liver damage. Am J Gastroenterol 1999;94(1):200–7.
51. Parks RW, Halliday MI, McCrory DC, et al. Host immune responses and intestinal permeability in patients with jaundice. Br J Surg 2003;90(2):239–45.
52. Shawcross DL, Wright GA, Stadlbauer V, et al. Ammonia impairs neutrophil phagocytic function in liver disease. Hepatology 2008;48(4):1202–12.
53. Koutelidakis I, Papaziogas B, Giamarellos-Bourboulis EJ, et al. Systemic endotoxaemia following obstructive jaundice: the role of lactulose. J Surg Res 2003;113(2):243–7.
54. Pain JA, Bailey ME. Experimental and clinical study of lactulose in obstructive jaundice. Br J Surg 1986;73(10):775–8.
55. Uslu A, Nart A, Colak T, et al. Predictors of mortality and morbidity in acute obstructive jaundice: implication of preventive measures. Hepatogastroenterology 2007;54(77):1331–4.

56. Freeman ML, Nelson DB, Sherman S, et al. Complications of endoscopic biliary sphincterotomy. N Engl J Med 1996;335(13):909–18.

57. Park DH, Kim MH, Lee SK, et al. Endoscopic sphincterotomy vs. endoscopic papillary balloon dilation for choledocholithiasis in patients with liver cirrhosis and coagulopathy. Gastrointest Endosc 2004;60(2):180–5.

58. Hayashida N, Shoujima T, Teshima H, et al. Clinical outcome after cardiac operations in patients with cirrhosis. Ann Thorac Surg 2004;77(2):500–5.

59. Suman A, Barnes DS, Zein NN, et al. Predicting outcome after cardiac surgery in patients with cirrhosis: a comparison of Child-Pugh and MELD scores. Clin Gastroenterol Hepatol 2004;2(8):719–23.

60. Semiz-Oysu A, Moustafa T, Cho KJ. Transjugular intrahepatic portosystemic shunt prior to cardiac surgery with cardiopulmonary bypass in patients with cirrhosis and portal hypertension. Heart Lung Circ 2007; 16(6):465–8.

61. Serfaty L, Aumaitre H, Chazouilleres O, et al. Determinants of outcome of compensated hepatitis C virus-related cirrhosis. Hepatology 1998;27(5):1435–40.

62. Fattovich G, Giustina G, Degos F, et al. Morbidity and mortality in compensated cirrhosis type C: a retrospective follow-up study of 384 patients. Gastroenterology 1997;112(2):463–72.

63. El-Serag HB. Hepatocellular carcinoma: recent trends in the United States. Gastroenterology 2004;127(5 Suppl 1):S27–34.

64. Bruix J, Sherman M. Management of hepatocellular carcinoma. Hepatology 2005; 42(5):1208–36.

65. Mullin EJ, Metcalfe MS, Maddern GJ. How much liver resection is too much? Am J Surg 2005;190(1):87–97.

66. Teh SH, Christein J, Donohue J, et al. Hepatic resection of hepatocellular carcinoma in patients with cirrhosis: Model of End-Stage Liver Disease (MELD) score predicts perioperative mortality. J Gastrointest Surg 2005;9(9): 1207–15.

67. Schroeder RA, Marroquin CE, Bute BP, et al. Predictive indices of morbidity and mortality after liver resection. Ann Surg 2006;243(3):373–9.

68. Cucchetti A, Ercolani G, Vivarelli M, et al. Impact of model for end-stage liver disease (MELD) score on prognosis after hepatectomy for hepatocellular carcinoma on cirrhosis. Liver Transpl 2006;12(6):966–71.

69. Hanazaki K, Kajikawa S, Koide N, et al. Prognostic factors after hepatic resection for hepatocellular carcinoma with hepatitis C viral infection: univariate and multivariate analysis. Am J Gastroenterol 2001;96(4):1243–50.

70. Nanashima A, Abo T, Sumida Y, et al. Clinicopathological characteristics of patients with hepatocellular carcinoma after hepatectomy: relationship with status of viral hepatitis. J Surg Oncol 2007;96(6):487–92.

71. Bellavance EC, Lumpkins KM, Mentha G, et al. Surgical management of early-stage hepatocellular carcinoma: resection or transplantation? J Gastrointest Surg 2008;12(10):1699–708.

72. Bigourdan JM, Jaeck D, Meyer N, et al. Small hepatocellular carcinoma in Child A cirrhotic patients: hepatic resection versus transplantation. Liver Transpl 2003; 9(5):513–20.

73. Schwartz M, Roayaie S, Uva P. Treatment of HCC in patients awaiting liver transplantation. Am J Transplant 2007;7(8):1875–81.

74. Cheng BQ, Jia CQ, Liu CT, et al. Chemoembolization combined with radiofrequency ablation for patients with hepatocellular carcinoma larger than 3 cm: a randomized controlled trial. JAMA 2008;299(14):1669–77.

75. Lodge JP, Jonas S, Jones RM, et al. Efficacy and safety of repeated perioperative doses of recombinant factor VIIa in liver transplantation. Liver Transpl 2005;11(8): 973–9.
76. Alkozai EM, Lisman T, Porte RJ. Bleeding in liver surgery: prevention and treatment. Clin Liver Dis 2009;13(1):145–54.
77. Marsman HA, Heisterkamp J, Halm JA, et al. Management in patients with liver cirrhosis and an umbilical hernia. Surgery 2007;142(3):372–5.
78. Fagan SP, Awad SS, Berger DH. Management of complicated umbilical hernias in patients with end-stage liver disease and refractory ascites. Surgery 2004;135(6): 679–82.
79. Arroyo V, Fernandez J, Gines P. Pathogenesis and treatment of hepatorenal syndrome. Semin Liver Dis 2008;28(1):81–95.
80. Duvoux C, Zanditenas D, Hezode C, et al. Effects of noradrenalin and albumin in patients with type I hepatorenal syndrome: a pilot study. Hepatology 2002;36(2): 374–80.
81. Wong F, Pantea L, Sniderman K. Midodrine, octreotide, albumin, and TIPS in selected patients with cirrhosis and type 1 hepatorenal syndrome. Hepatology 2004;40(1):55–64.
82. Cordoba J, Minguez B. Hepatic encephalopathy. Semin Liver Dis 2008;28(1):70–80.
83. Lawrence KR, Klee JA. Rifaximin for the treatment of hepatic encephalopathy. Pharmacotherapy 2008;28(8):1019–32.
84. Garcia-Tsao G, Sanyal AJ, Grace ND, et al. Prevention and management of gastroesophageal varices and variceal hemorrhage in cirrhosis. Hepatology 2007;46(3):922–38.
85. Campillo B, Bories PN, Pornin B, et al. Influence of liver failure, ascites, and energy expenditure on the response to oral nutrition in alcoholic liver cirrhosis. Nutrition 1997;13(7-8):613–21.
86. Tsiaousi ET, Hatzitolios AI, Trygonis SK, et al. Malnutrition in end stage liver disease: recommendations and nutritional support. J Gastroenterol Hepatol 2008;23(4):527–33.
87. Merli M, Nicolini G, Angeloni S, et al. Malnutrition is a risk factor in cirrhotic patients undergoing surgery. Nutrition 2002;18(11–12):978–86.
88. Poulsen TL, Thulstrup AM, Sorensen HT, et al. Appendicectomy and perioperative mortality in patients with liver cirrhosis. Br J Surg 2000;87(12):1664–5.
89. Gervaz P, Pak-art R, Nivatvongs S, et al. Colorectal adenocarcinoma in cirrhotic patients. J Am Coll Surg 2003;196(6):874–9.
90. Tachibana M, Kotoh T, Kinugasa S, et al. Esophageal cancer with cirrhosis of the liver: results of esophagectomy in 18 consecutive patients. Ann Surg Oncol 2000; 7(10):758–63.
91. Shih LY, Cheng CY, Chang CH, et al. Total knee arthroplasty in patients with liver cirrhosis. J Bone Joint Surg Am 2004;86-A(2):335–41.
92. Milanez de Campos JR, Filho LO, de Campos Werebe E, et al. Thoracoscopy and talc poudrage in the management of hepatic hydrothorax. Chest 2000;118(1): 13–7.

Modern Diagnosis and Management of Hepatocellular Carcinoma

Jorge A. Marrero, MD, MS[a],*, Theodore Welling, MD[b]

KEYWORDS

- Liver cancer • Cirrhosis • Hepatitis C
- Hepatitis B • Surveillance

Hepatocellular carcinoma (HCC) is one of the commonest solid malignancies world-wide,[1] with an increasing incidence in the United States.[2] Over the last 10 years, it has had the second highest increase in incidence and one of the highest increases in death rate in the United States.[3] It has been estimated that the number of cases of HCC will continue to increase by 81% (from a baseline of about 13,000 a year) by the year 2020, predominantly due to hepatitis C (HCV) infection. Despite advances in medical technology, the 5-year survival between 1981 and 1998 improved only 3%, reflecting that most patients with HCC are diagnosed at more advanced stages, leading to an overall 1-year survival of 25% in the United States.[4] In this setting of a significant increase in the number of patients with HCC, early detection and treatment of this tumor are vital to improve outcomes.

EARLY DETECTION

Screening has been shown to be effective in enhancing survival in patients with breast, colon, and cervical cancers.[5] Although the overall goal is to reduce morbidity and mortality from cancer, the objective of screening is the use of a simple, inexpensive test on a large number of individuals to determine whether they are likely or unlikely to have the cancer for which they are being screened.[6] Screening is the one-time application of a test that allows detection of asymptomatic disease at a stage when curative intervention may improve the goal of reducing morbidity and mortality.

This work was supported by DK64909 and DK077707 (JAM).

[a] Division of Gastroenterology, Department of Internal Medicine, University of Michigan, 3912 Taubman Center, Ann Arbor, MI 48109-0362, USA
[b] Division of Transplant, Department of Surgery, University of Michigan, 2926F Taubman Center, Ann Arbor, MI 48109-0331, USA
* Corresponding author.
E-mail address: jmarrero@umich.edu (J.A. Marrero).

Clin Liver Dis 13 (2009) 233–247
doi:10.1016/j.cld.2009.02.007
1089-3261/09/$ – see front matter © 2009 Elsevier Inc. All rights reserved.

Surveillance is the continuous monitoring of disease occurrence (using the screening test) within a population to achieve the same goals as screening. Criteria have been developed, first promoted by the World Health Organization, to ensure the benefits of screening or surveillance for a specific disease:[7] (1) the disease in question should be an important health problem; its significance may be defined by disease burden, including morbidity and mortality; (2) there should be an identifiable target population; (3) treatment of occult disease (ie, disease diagnosed before the symptoms appear) should offer advantages compared with the treatment of symptomatic disease; (4) a screening test should be affordable and provide benefits justifying its cost; (5) the test must be acceptable to the target population and to health care professionals; (6) there must be standardized recall procedures; and (7) screening tests must achieve an acceptable level of accuracy in the population undergoing screening. HCC meets all of these criteria for establishment of a surveillance program. Before developing a surveillance program, it is critical to decide what level of risk for HCC is significant enough to warrant initiation of surveillance, what screening tests are to be applied and at what frequency, and how abnormal results from screening tests (diagnosis or recall) are dealt with.

Several decision analysis models have shown that surveillance for HCC is a cost-effective strategy[8–10] and indicate that an incidence rate of HCC of at least 1.5% per annum should trigger surveillance. Patients at risk for HCC should be divided into those with hepatitis B (HBV) and those without HBV. The risk of HCC in patients with chronic HBV infection will depend on age, carrier status, inflammation, family history of HCC, and the presence or absence of cirrhosis.[11] Prospective studies have shown that the annual incidence rate of HCC in patients with HBV cirrhosis is between 2.2% and 4.3%, ranging from 0.1% to 1% in patients with chronic hepatitis and 0.02% to 0.2% in inactive carriers.[12] **Box 1** describes the patients with chronic HBV infection for whom surveillance is recommended. For those without chronic HBV infection, the risk for developing HCC, and therefore the group in which surveillance is recommended, is limited to those with cirrhosis, as shown in **Box 1**. The annual incidence rate for patients with HCV-related HCC is 3.7% to 7.1%, and 0.2% to 1.8% for those with alcohol-related cirrhosis.[12] There are no large prospective studies to determine the incidence of HCC for other causes of cirrhosis, but their risk is significantly elevated compared with the normal population.

As the goal of screening is to reduce mortality by detecting patients with occult disease, the performance characteristics of a test used for diagnosis or staging (eg, computed tomography (CT) or MRI) cannot be assumed to be the same when used in a surveillance/screening situation. The most commonly used screening test for HCC is serum alpha-fetoprotein (AFP). It has been shown that the optimal balance of sensitivity and specificity is achieved by a cutoff level of 20 ng/mL.[13] However, this cutoff leads to sensitivities between 41% and 60% and specificities between 80% and 94%.[14–16] The other frequently used test for surveillance is abdominal ultrasound (US). The sensitivity of US has been shown to be between 58% and 78% and the specificity between 93% and 98%.[17–19] However, the performance characteristics of US as a surveillance test for HCC have been extrapolated mostly from studies that evaluated US as a diagnostic test, and therefore its performance as a surveillance test has not been definitively established. One of the major problems of the prospective cohort studies assessing the performance of AFP and US in surveillance for HCC is the poor sample size in published studies. Pooling the number of patients in studies that evaluated AFP and US as screening tests for HCC only shows a total sample size of about 19,000 (only 1,000 in studies with patients with cirrhosis). In contrast, more than 200,000 patients were involved separately in the evaluation of screening

Box 1
High-risk groups for hepatocellular carcinoma
Hepatitis B carriers
Asian men older than 40 years
Asian women older than 50 years
Cirrhosis
Family history of hepatocellular carcinoma
Noncirrhotics: depends on viral genotype, viral replication, inflammatory activity
Nonhepatitis B cirrhosis
Hepatitis C
Alcohol
Hereditary hemochromatosis
Primary biliary cirrhosis
Not enough evidence for the following:
α-1 antitrypsin deficiency
Non–alcohol-related fatty liver disease
Autoimmune hepatitis
Adapted from Bruix J, Sherman M. Management of hepatocellular carcinoma. Hepatology 2005;42:1208–36; with permission.

tests for breast, colon, and cervical cancers.[20–22] Other important limitations of studies evaluating surveillance tests for HCC are the lack of assessment of the performance of a definitive test to detect occult disease, and the absence of studies in cirrhotic patients linking surveillance performance with outcomes. Furthermore, the performance of US is operator dependent. The recent guidelines of the American Association for the Study of Liver Disease recommended surveillance with US with a level II recommendation, based on case–control or uncontrolled cohort studies, and at a frequency of 6 to 12 months.[11] However, further studies are needed to truly assess the performance of AFP and US as surveillance tests in patients with cirrhosis.

A recent randomized controlled study of screening for HCC has been reported from China.[23] This study compared US and AFP versus no screening. It achieved a compliance rate of less than 60% and found that screening led to a reduction of 37% in mortality compared with no screening. One limitation of this study is that only patients with HBV infection, remote or current, were enrolled and therefore not all the patients had the same risk level of developing HCC. Another limitation is that, because of the low compliance rate with screening in this study, it may have underestimated the benefits of surveillance. However, this is the first evidence that surveillance for HCC with AFP and US improves mortality. Additional randomized trials of screening for HCC are needed in other geographic areas and cirrhotic populations to confirm the benefits of screening.

DIAGNOSIS

Once an abnormality is detected on a screening test, a recall test is performed to determine the presence of HCC. For the diagnosis of HCC, a radiologic test, such as triple-phase spiral CT, dynamic MRI, biopsy, or significantly elevated AFP, are the diagnostic tests of choice. A recent prospective study showed that MRI has a sensitivity and specificity of 75% and 76%, respectively, with a likelihood ratio of 3:1 for a diagnosis of HCC, which is superior to a sensitivity and specificity of 61% and 66%, respectively, for triple-phase spiral CT, with a likelihood ratio of 1:8.[24] Other studies have confirmed that MRI is slightly superior to CT scanning for definitive diagnosis of HCC.[25,26] The major finding on CT and MRI that suggests HCC is an arterially enhancing lesion in the liver of a patient with cirrhosis.[27] However, recent studies suggest that not only arterial enhancement of a hepatic nodule is important but also washout of contrast in the delayed phases of enhancement. Washout is defined as hypointensity of a nodule in delayed phases of CT or MRI examination compared with surrounding liver parenchyma.[28] It is likely due to arterial neovascularization and is greater in HCC nodules than in the surrounding nonneoplastic hepatic parenchyma, and in delayed phases there is early venous drainage.[29] The presence of washout in an arterially enhancing lesion increases the probability of HCC 65-fold.[30] Arterial enhancement with washout of a mass in a cirrhotic liver has a sensitivity of about 80% but a specificity of 95% to 100%. If a lesion does not meet these criteria, then a liver biopsy should be performed if AFP is not markedly elevated. The diagnostic workup of a patient with an abnormal surveillance test for HCC is shown in **Fig. 1**, as recommended by the HCC guidelines of the American Association for the Study of Liver Disease.[11]

Tumor nodules less than 2 cm in size are difficult to characterize and the performance of MRI or CT is significantly worse compared with larger lesions, and therefore biopsy may be necessary.[11,31] However, even histologic examination may not be diagnostic, especially as there is a lack of novel markers to aid in differentiation of small HCC from dysplastic nodules.[11] Recent molecular advances have shown that a 3-gene set incorporating glypican-3, surviving and lymphatic vessel endothelial hyaluronan receptor-1 (LYVE1) improved the ability to differentiate early HCC from dysplastic nodules.[31] Glypican-3 (18-fold increase in HCC, $P = .01$), LYVE1 (12-fold decrease in HCC, $P = .0001$), and survivin (2.2-fold increase in HCC, $P = .02$) had a discriminative accuracy of 94%. Glypican-3 use was confirmed in another study to help in differentiating small HCCs from dysplastic nodules on histologic analysis.[32] It seems consistent that glypican-3 does improve the ability to diagnose HCC at an early stage.

TREATMENT

A variety of HCC therapies are discussed with emphasis on expected survival rates and overall indications. It should be emphasized that, whereas in many instances one therapy may appear superior to another, treatment must be individualized. Individualized treatment is particularly relevant for possible side effects of therapies, patients with underlying liver disease, tumor characteristics, and overall patient performance status. Therapeutic goals of the modalities vary from potentially curative to palliative, and from directed therapy to systemic therapy. Overall survival represents the standard by which to judge most therapies because this measure reflects the overall burden of tumor stage, liver disease, and the complications of therapies. The Barcelona Clinic Liver Cancer (BCLC) staging system is considered to be the most accurate predictive system in decision making regarding therapies, incorporating existing liver disease, tumor stage, and overall performance status.[33] This staging system has been independently validated in separate studies evaluating therapeutic outcomes in HCC patients and has been found to be more predictive than older staging systems.[34] The BCLC staging system is shown in **Fig. 2**.

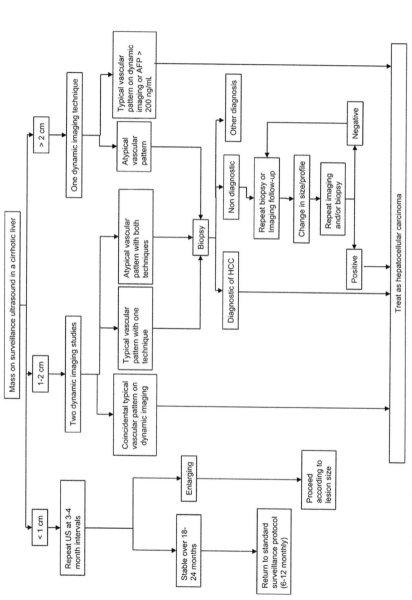

Fig. 1. Algorithm for the evaluation of an abnormal liver ultrasound or α-fetoprotein for patients with HCC. The typical vascular pattern referred to means that the lesion is hypervascular in the arterial phase, and washes out in the portal/venous phase. All other patterns are considered atypical. (*From* Bruix J, Sherman M. Management of hepatocellular carcinoma. Hepatology 2005;42:1208–36; with permission.)

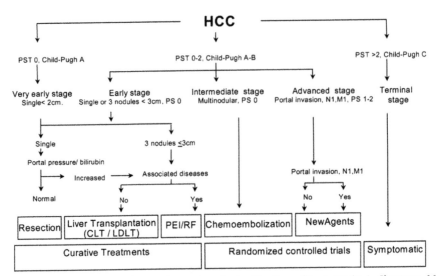

Fig. 2. The Barcelona staging and treatment classification. (*From* Bruix J, Sherman M. Management of hepatocellular carcinoma. Hepatology 2005;42:1208–36; with permission.)

Hepatic Resection

Hepatic resection is the treatment of choice for patients with HCC without cirrhosis. There is no size limit for patients without cirrhosis, but for those with cirrhosis, resection leads to better outcomes among those with BCLC very early stage (tumors <2 cm without portal hypertension) or selected patients at BCLC stage A (tumors <5 cm without portal hypertension). When patients are properly selected, survival rates approach 38% to 70% at 5 years with disease-free survival ranging from 28% to 54.8% in case series and multicenter databases.[35–37] Perioperative mortality rates are generally on the order of 4.0% to 4.7% for resections for HCC,[38] which contrasts with mortality rates of 0.0% to 0.9% for resections for benign disease or colorectal metastasis,[39–41] and reflects associated chronic liver disease in patients with HCC. Selection of patients is critical and depends on the following factors: degree of hepatic fibrosis, planned future liver remnant, tumor characteristics, patient performance status, and whether patients will benefit similarly from other treatments, such as liver transplantation or radiofrequency ablation (RFA).

The degree of hepatic function clearly impacts survival following resection as evaluated by model for end-stage liver disease (MELD) or Child–Pugh scores. Patients with a Child's B score or greater, although they have an appreciable survival rate at 5 years of 20% to 50%, have decreased survival compared with Child's A patients that approaches the survival rate of ablative therapies for tumors of similar size.[42–44] In addition, patients with MELD scores of greater than 9 have high mortality rates following resection (29%) making other therapies more attractive.[45] Other markers of significant portal hypertension (platelet count <100,000/mm^3 or hepatic vein pressure gradient >10 mmHg) have been used to assess surgical risk and remain a relative exclusion to surgical therapy in most centers.[46] Case series have established that a planned small future liver remnant of less than 40% of total liver volume contributes to mortality in patients with chronic liver disease.[47] Therefore, assessment of the presence of liver disease and planned future liver remnant are critical for determining the eligibility of patients for resection. Patients with a decreased planned liver remnant are eligible for preoperative portal vein embolization on the portion planned for resection to allow compensatory hypertrophy of the unaffected side, resulting in an increase in the planned future liver remnant. Centers of excellence performing these maneuvers have shown a reduction in complications related to hepatic dysfunction, as well as the ability to recruit more patients for resection although no randomized trials exist.

The success of surgical therapy has also been related to tumor characteristics. Tumor size, tumor number, and the presence of macro- or microvascular invasion have been noted to correlate with a reduction in survival postresection.[37,47] The most important factor is vascular invasion with a reduction in 5-year survival from 41% to 57% down to 15% to 34.5% in 2 multi-institutional studies.[48] Whereas tumor size is linked to poorer outcomes, this is believed to be linked primarily to vascular invasion as tumor size is noted to correlate directly with the incidence of vascular invasion.[48] However, patients with extremely large HCCs, often presenting without cirrhosis or vascular invasion, can have 5-year survival rates postresection of as high as 54% to 57.7%[49,50] but these rates diminish by half if cirrhosis or vascular invasion are present. Of the other variables that have been evaluated to provide prognostic information, the most important is AFP level. AFP levels have been shown to correlate directly with the presence of vascular invasion, with AFP levels greater than 1,000 ng/mL in one study[51,52] and greater than 200 ng/mL in another[53] associated with vascular invasion in 61% of patients.

Some degree of controversy exists about the management of HCCs less than 2.0 cm in diameter. A randomized controlled trial evaluating RFA versus resection revealed equivalent results (4-year survival of 64% with RFA vs. 67.9% with resection, P = NS) with the overall attendant reduction in periprocedure risk that accompanies RFA when compared with resection.[53] Therefore, location of small tumors and the presence or absence of chronic liver disease and portal hypertension dictates the choice of therapy selection (RFA vs resection).

As HCC is known to recur in 70% of patients within 5 years postresection, with most of these occurrences after 2 years,[35,54,55] there has been considerable interest in developing adjuvant therapies following resection. No adjuvant therapy with proven efficacy for HCC postresection exists currently. An early randomized controlled trial evaluating interferon showed initial positive results in limiting recurrence.[56] However, a more recent study showed limited benefit with some efficacy for patients with hepatitis B-related cirrhosis and more advanced HCC tumors (pathological tumor-node-metastasis stage III/IVA) by increasing the 5-year survival from 24% to 68%.[57] Molecular targeted therapies offer great potential as adjuvant therapies to prevent recurrence.

Laparoscopic liver resection is gaining favor at a variety of centers as surgical technologies continue to evolve. The most encouraging report was a matched case series with reported reductions in length of stay, decreased blood loss, and decreased complications in select cases.[58] However, this and other experiences represent highly selected patients. Similar to other fields in which laparoscopy has been used, additional benefits for a laparoscopic approach will likely be described in the near future.

Liver Transplantation

Liver transplantation offers the ability to treat HCC, the underlying liver disease, and in theory limit recurrences by treating the liver disease. Following the pivotal study by Mazzaferro and colleagues,[59] liver transplantation has been an accepted therapy for HCC, especially in patients who are not eligible for liver resection and qualify for listing based on the Milan staging system, originally applied in this study. This study showed that a 4-year survival rate of 75% was achievable and this rose to 85% when patients who had pathology consistent with the preoperative imaging were analyzed. The Milan criterion for transplant is for single tumors less than or equal to 5.0 cm or 2 to 3 tumors with the largest less than or equal to 3.0 cm, but some groups suggest that this is too restrictive. The University of California at San Francisco (UCSF) has proposed expansion of the criterion to a tumor size less than or equal to 6.5 cm or 2 to 3 tumors (none >4.5 cm) and have reported a 5-year survival rate of 88.5%.[60] The data to date have revealed mixed results,[61,62] and more studies are needed to determine the applicability of expanding the criteria for transplant.

In an effort to achieve relative equality for a scarce resource, an allocation system has been devised so that HCC patients meeting the Milan criteria qualify for MELD exception points, to minimize waitlist dropouts due to disease progression and at the same time not to divert too many donor livers away from the remainder of the recipient candidate pool. In the latest review of outcomes and patterns of liver transplantation for patients with HCC as reported by the Scientific Registry of Transplant Recipients (SRTR),[63] some interesting trends are noted. During the MELD era, the adjusted 3-year survival rate for HCC patients was 74%, statistically lower than non-HCC recipients (81%). Five-year survival data for HCC patients treated with transplantation during the MELD era are not yet available. The role of bridging therapy or neoadjuvant therapy with ablative techniques such as RFA remains controversial for liver transplant patients. Although this latest SRTR report indicates that patients treated with such therapy had a 3-year survival rate of 79% versus 75% ($P = .03$) compared with HCC patients who were not treated, limited numbers of patients and obvious selection bias limit the interpretation of the use of this practice. Randomized trials are required to firmly determine the role and application of bridging therapy. There does appear to be a role for downstaging of tumors that are just outside the Milan criteria. Using RFA or transarterial chemoembolization (TACE), downstaging is possible in as many as 70% of patients, with 2-year survival of 81% following transplantation and a median time of about 8 months after the downstaging therapy has been performed.[64]

Besides the overall influence of tumor size, other prognostic factors have been evaluated for their effects on outcomes of transplantation for HCC. In particular, multivariate single center analyses have shown that, similar to resection outcomes, the presence of vascular invasion or AFP greater than 300 ng/mL are negative prognostic factors.[65,66] In a recent retrospective series comparing resection to transplantation, tumors meeting the Milan criteria had equal 5-year survival with resection or transplantation when stratified for the absence of vascular invasion, making it less clear whether transplantation was superior to resection.[67] Therefore, improved methods to accurately determine the presence of vascular invasion are especially needed for purposes of screening before transplantation.

Locoregional Therapies

Many locoregional therapies have been proposed for the treatment of HCC and have included cryoablation, percutaneous ethanol ablation (PEA), microwave ablation, RFA, TACE, radiotherapy, and yttrium-90 microspheres. Of the ablative therapies, RFA has emerged as the treatment of choice when compared with cryoablation and PEA.[68] Randomized controlled studies in Asia on tumors less than 4.0 cm in size have shown superior survival benefit of RFA over PEA with 4-year survival of 74% achieved with RFA.[69,70] In addition, RFA seems to be most beneficial for tumors less than 3.0 cm in size with efficacy decreasing as larger tumors are treated. Based on response rates analyzed by posttreatment imaging, RFA achieves a greater rate of tumor necrosis

(70% for tumors 2–3 cm in size) than PEA and often with less sessions or treatments required. Compared to microwave therapy, RFA has also been tested in a randomized controlled trial with both showing equivalent results and complication rates. However, a greater number of treatment sessions were required for microwave therapy.[68] Cryotherapy is one of the older ablation therapies, but results have been less favorable with 3- and 5-year survival rates of 40.3% and 26.9%, respectively.[71] In addition, the complication rate of cryotherapy is believed to be higher than RFA with hemorrhage and coagulation abnormalities being more common.[72]

As discussed earlier, a randomized controlled trial has compared RFA with resection for small HCCs (<2.0 cm) and suggested that these 2 modalities are equivalent.[53] Contrary to this finding, the Japanese Nationwide survey of HCCs, which evaluated patients with less than Milan stage II tumors and greater than 2,500 patients in each group, found that there was a decreased incidence of recurrence at 2 years in the resection group.[73] Although these findings need to be confirmed in other trials, RFA offers a potential therapeutic option to patients otherwise unfit for surgery.

TACE has been evaluated in several randomized controlled studies. A recent meta-analysis of these trials showed an improved 2-year survival with an odds ratio of 0.53 (95% confidence interval, 0.32–0.89, $P = .17$) when TACE was compared with best supportive care, translating to a median survival increase of 16 months to 20 months.[74] The best results for TACE are on patients at the BCLC intermediate stage. Therefore, TACE is believed to be an option for patients who are not otherwise candidates for resection, transplant, or RFA. In one of the largest prospective cohort studies, median survival was noted to be 34 months with a 5-year survival of 26%.[74–76] The roles of doxorubicin or cisplatin as part of the TACE regimen remain uncertain, but they have shown benefit in at least 2 different randomized trials.[54,55] Relative contraindications to the use of TACE are essentially portal vein thrombosis or more overt hepatic insufficiency with many Child's B and all Child's C patients unsuitable as candidates due to the risk of inducing hepatocellular failure.

Other locoregional therapies are being studied. These modalities have been primarily evaluated in single center case series. Yttrium-90 microspheres have received the most attention recently at several centers as a means of achieving microscopic brachytherapy to the well-vascularized HCC tumor. The largest experience evaluated 209 patients with advanced HCC with 42.2% of patients achieving a partial response and a median survival of 12 months.[77] These studies included patients at the BCLC intermediate stage and advanced stage, both of which have different natural history, and therefore it is hard to determine its true efficacy. External beam radiotherapy has been used in patients not otherwise eligible for other locoregional therapies or resection and included patients with T1 to T4 lesions.[78] Larger studies are needed to determine the role, efficacy, and safety of external radiotherapy for patients with HCC. Finally, doxorubicin eluting beads have also been studied for safety with a response rate of 75% in treated patients.[79]

Systemic Therapy

Several agents have been investigated as systemic therapy for HCC in randomized controlled trials.[80] These agents have essentially no efficacy in treating HCC when compared with appropriate controls and have included tamoxifen, doxorubicin, combination cisplatin/interferon α2b/doxorubicin/fluorouracil, seocalcitol, nolatrexed, and a tubulin inhibitor.

Directed molecular therapies have evolved for the treatment of other cancer sites including breast, colon, and renal cells. The most promising agent for HCC, sorafenib, has been studied in a randomized controlled trial of patients with advanced disease.[81] This agent has activity against tyrosine kinases such as the vascular endothelial growth factor (VEGF) receptor 2, the platelet-derived growth factor receptor, and c-kit receptors and also has activity against serine/threonine kinases (b-Raf/Ras/MAPKK pathway). Thus, cell proliferation and angiogenesis are inhibited by sorafenib. The SHARP trial evaluated 299 patients in the sorafenib group versus 303 in the control group and demonstrated a significant increase in median survival from 7.9 months to 10.7 months (hazard ratio, 0.58, 95% confidence interval, 0.45–0.74) as shown in **Fig. 3**. Sorafenib also delayed the time to progression from 2.8 months in the placebo group to 5.5 months (P < .001). Overall this therapy was well tolerated with most side effects being mild to moderate in severity; only 8% of patients suffered grade 3 toxicities (diarrhea or hand–foot skin reaction). Thus, sorafenib represents the first line therapy for patients with advanced HCC.

Whether sorafenib will have other roles in the treatment of HCC is the subject of current trial designs. For example, sorafenib may have benefit when used as an adjuvant to resection, ablation, or other locoregional therapies. In addition, many agents have recently been or are currently in phase II studies: bevacizumab (VEGF inhibitor), sunitinib (multityrosine kinase inhibitor), erlotinib (EGF receptor inhibitor), and gefitinib (EGF receptor inhibitor).[80]

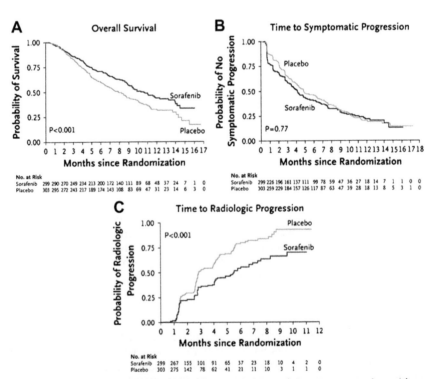

Fig. 3. Overall survival, time to symptomatic progression and time to progression with sorafenib for advanced hepatocellular carcinoma. (*From* Llovet JM, Ricci S, Mazzaferro V, et al. Sorafenib in advanced hepatocellular carcinoma. N Engl J Med 2008;359:378–90; with permission.)

SUMMARY

Surgical resection or transplantation represents the best chance for overall survival in selected patients. Other modalities such as RFA offer reasonable alternatives and survival probability for patients who are otherwise not candidates for surgery or transplantation. Therapies such as TACE and sorafenib offer significant survival benefit for more advanced tumors. Multimodality or combined approaches are currently under investigation and represent additional hope for improved efficacy against HCC in the future.

REFERENCES

1. Parkin DM, Bray F, Ferlay J, et al. Estimating the world cancer burden: Globocan 2000. Int J Cancer 2001;94:153–6.
2. El Serag HB, Mason AC. Rising incidence of hepatocellular carcinoma in the United States. N Engl J Med 1999;340:745–50.
3. El-Serag HB, Davila JA, Petersen NJ, et al. The continuing increase in the incidence of hepatocellular carcinoma in the United States: an update. Ann Intern Med 2003;139(10):817–23.
4. El Serag HB, Mason AC, Key C. Trends in survival of patients with hepatocellular carcinoma between 1977 and 1996 in the United States. Hepatology 2001;33: 62–5.
5. Meissner HI, Smith RA, Rimer BK, et al. Promoting cancer screening: learning from experience. Cancer 2004;101:1107–17.
6. Smith RA. Screening fundamentals. J Natl Cancer Inst Monogr 1997;22:15–9.
7. Cole P, Morrison AS. Basic issues in population screening for cancer. J Natl Cancer Inst 1980;64:1263–72.
8. Sarasin FP, Giostra E, Hadengue A. Cost-effectiveness of screening for detection of small hepatocellular carcinoma in western patients with Child-Pugh class A cirrhosis. Am J Med 1996;101:422–34.
9. Arguedas MR, Chen VK, Eloubeidi MA, et al. Screening for hepatocellular carcinoma in patients with hepatitis C cirrhosis: a cost-utility analysis. Am J Gastroenterol 2003;98:679–90.
10. Lin OS, Keeffe EB, Sanders GD, et al. Cost-effectiveness of screening for hepatocellular carcinoma in patients with cirrhosis due to chronic hepatitis C. Aliment Pharmacol Ther 2004;19:1159–72.
11. Bruix J, Sherman M. Management of hepatocellular carcinoma. Hepatology 2005; 42:1208–36.
12. Fattovich G, Stroffollini T, Zagne I, et al. Hepatocellular carcinoma in cirrhosis: incidence and risk factors. Gastroenterology 2004;127:S35–50.
13. Trevisani F, D'Intino PE, Morselli-Labate AM, et al. Serum alpha-fetoprotein for diagnosis of hepatocellular carcinoma in patients with chronic liver disease: influence of HBsAg and anti-HCV status. J Hepatol 2001;34:570–5.
14. Marrero JA. Screening tests for hepatocellular carcinoma. Clin Liver Dis 2005;9: 235–51.
15. Pateron D, Ganne N, Trinchet JC, et al. Prospective study of screening for hepatocellular carcinoma in Caucasian patients with cirrhosis. J Hepatol 1994;20: 65–71.
16. Zoli M, Magalotti D, Bianchi G, et al. Efficacy of a surveillance program for early detection of hepatocellular carcinoma. Cancer 1996;78:977–85.

17. Chen TH, Chen CJ, Yen MF, et al. Ultrasound screening and risk factors for death from hepatocellular carcinoma in a high risk group in Taiwan. Int J Cancer 2002; 98:257–61.
18. Larcos G, Sorokopud H, Berry G, et al. Sonographic screening for hepatocellular carcinoma in patients with chronic hepatitis or cirrhosis: an evaluation. AJR Am J Roentgenol 1998;171:433–5.
19. Zhang B, Yang B. Combined alpha fetoprotein testing and ultrasonography as a screening test for primary liver cancer. J Med Screen 1999;6:108–10.
20. Ransohoff DF. Colon cancer screening in 2005: status and challenges. Gastroenterology 2005;128:1685–95.
21. Smith RA, Saslow D, Andrews-Sawyer K, et al. American Cancer Society guidelines for breast cancer screening: update 2003. CA Cancer J Clin 2003;53:141–69.
22. Saslow D, Runowicz CD, Solomon C, et al. American Cancer Society guideline for the early detection of cervical neoplasia and cancer. CA Cancer J Clin 2002;52: 342–62.
23. Zhang BH, Yang BH, Tang ZY. Randomized controlled trial of screening for hepatocellular carcinoma. J Cancer Res Clin Oncol 2004;130:417–22.
24. Burrel M, Llovet JM, Ayuso C, et al. MRI angiography is superior to helical CT for detection of HCC prior to liver transplantation: an explant correlation. Hepatology 2003;38:1034–42.
25. Krinsky GA, Lee VS, Thiese ND, et al. Hepatocellular carcinoma and dysplastic nodules in patients with cirrhosis: prospective diagnosis with MR imaging and explant correlation. Radiology 2001;219:445–54.
26. Rode A, Bancel B, Douek P, et al. Small nodule detection in cirrhotic livers: evaluation with US, spiral CT and MRI and correlation with pathologic examination of explanted liver. J Comput Assist Tomogr 2001;25:327–36.
27. Bruix J, Sherman M, Llovet JM, et al. Clinical management of hepatocellular carcinoma: conclusions of the Barcelona-2000 EASL conference. J Hepatol 2001;35:421–30.
28. Hayashi M, Matsui O, Ueda K, et al. Progression to hypervascular hepatocellular carcinoma: correlation with intranodular blood supply evaluated with CT during intraarterial injection of contrast material. Radiology 2002;225:143–9.
29. Lim JH, Kim EY, Lee WJ, et al. Regenerative nodules in liver cirrhosis: findings at CT during arterial portography and CT hepatic arteriography with histopathologic correlation. Radiology 1999;210:451–8.
30. Marrero JA, Hussain HK, Umar RK, et al. Improving the prediction of hepatocellular carcinoma in cirrhotics with an arterially enhancing liver mass. Liver Transpl 2005;11:281–9.
31. Llovet JM, Chen Y, Wurmbach E, et al. A molecular signature to discriminate dysplastic nodules from early hepatocellular carcinoma in HCV cirrhosis. Gastroenterology 2006;131(6):1758–67.
32. Libbrecht L, Severi T, Cassiman D, et al. Glypican-3 expression distinguishes small hepatocellular carcinomas from cirrhosis, dysplastic nodules, and focal nodular hyperplasia-like nodules. Am J Surg Pathol 2006;30(11):1405–11.
33. Llovet JM, Bru C, Bruix J. Prognosis of hepatocellular carcinoma: the BCLC staging classification. Semin Liver Dis 1999;19:329–38.
34. Marrero JA, Fontana RJ, Barrat A, et al. Prognosis of hepatocellular carcinoma: comparison of 7 staging systems in an American cohort. Hepatology 2005;41:707–16.
35. Chang CH, Chau GY, Lui WY, et al. Long-term results of hepatic resection for hepatocellular carcinoma originating from the noncirrhotic liver. Arch Surg 2004;139:320–5.

36. Cho CS, Gonen M, Shia J, et al. A novel prognostic nomogram is more accurate than conventional staging systems for predicting survival after resection of hepatocellular carcinoma. J Am Coll Surg 2008;206:281–91.

37. Vauthey JN, Lauwers GY, Esnaola NF, et al. Simplified staging for hepatocellular carcinoma. J Clin Oncol 2002;20:1527–36.

38. Asiyanbola B, Chang D, Gleisner AL, et al. Operative mortality after hepatic resection: are literature-based rates broadly applicable? J Gastrointest Surg 2008;12:842–51.

39. Parikh AA, Gentner B, Wu TT, et al. Perioperative complications in patients undergoing major liver resection with or without neoadjuvant chemotherapy. J Gastrointest Surg 2003;7:1082–8.

40. Pawlik TM, Scoggins CR, Zorzi D, et al. Effect of surgical margin status on survival and site of recurrence after hepatic resection for colorectal metastases. Ann Surg 2005;241:715–22.

41. Cho SW, Marsh JW, Steel J, et al. Surgical management of hepatocellular adenoma: take it or leave it? Ann Surg Oncol 2008;15:2795–803.

42. Wayne JD, Lauwers GY, Ikai I, et al. Preoperative predictors of survival after resection of small hepatocellular carcinomas. Ann Surg 2002;235:722–30 [discussion: 730–1].

43. Tateishi R, Shiina S, Teratani T, et al. Percutaneous radiofrequency ablation for hepatocellular carcinoma. An analysis of 1000 cases. Cancer 2005;103:1201–9.

44. Arii S, Yamaoka Y, Futagawa S, et al. Results of surgical and nonsurgical treatment for small-sized hepatocellular carcinomas: a retrospective and nationwide survey in Japan. The Liver Cancer Study Group of Japan. Hepatology 2000;32:1224–9.

45. Teh SH, Christein J, Donohue J, et al. Hepatic resection of hepatocellular carcinoma in patients with cirrhosis: model of end-stage liver disease (MELD) score predicts perioperative mortality. J Gastrointest Surg 2005;9:1207–15.

46. Bruix J, Castells A, Bosch J, et al. Surgical resection of hepatocellular carcinoma in cirrhotic patients: prognostic value of preoperative portal pressure. Gastroenterology 1996;111:1018–22.

47. Farges O, Belghiti J, Kianmanesh R, et al. Portal vein embolization before right hepatectomy: prospective clinical trial. Ann Surg 2003;237:208–17.

48. Pawlik TM, Delman KA, Vauthey JN, et al. Tumor size predicts vascular invasion and histologic grade: implications for selection of surgical treatment for hepatocellular carcinoma. Liver Transpl 2005;11:1086–92.

49. Pandey D, Lee KH, Wai CT, et al. Long term outcome and prognostic factors for large hepatocellular carcinoma (10 cm or more) after surgical resection. Ann Surg Oncol 2007;14:2817–23.

50. Shah SA, Wei AC, Cleary SP, et al. Prognosis and results after resection of very large (≥10 cm) hepatocellular carcinoma. J Gastrointest Surg 2007;11:589–95.

51. Sakata J, Shirai Y, Wakai T, et al. Preoperative predictors of vascular invasion in hepatocellular carcinoma. Eur J Surg Oncol 2008;34:900–5.

52. Peng SY, Chen WJ, Lai PL, et al. High alpha-fetoprotein level correlates with high stage, early recurrence and poor prognosis of hepatocellular carcinoma: significance of hepatitis virus infection, age, p53 and beta-catenin mutations. Int J Cancer 2004;112:44–50.

53. Chen MS, Li JQ, Zheng Y, et al. A prospective randomized trial comparing percutaneous local ablative therapy and partial hepatectomy for small hepatocellular carcinoma. Ann Surg 2006;243:321–8.

54. Poon RT, Fan ST, Lo CM, et al. Long-term survival and pattern of recurrence after resection of small hepatocellular carcinoma in patients with preserved liver

function: implications for a strategy of salvage transplantation. Ann Surg 2002; 235:373–82.

55. Kumada T, Nakano S, Takeda I, et al. Patterns of recurrence after initial treatment in patients with small hepatocellular carcinoma. Hepatology 1997;25:87–92.

56. Kubo S, Nishiguchi S, Hirohashi K, et al. Effects of long-term postoperative interferon-alpha therapy on intrahepatic recurrence after resection of hepatitis C virus-related hepatocellular carcinoma. A randomized, controlled trial. Ann Intern Med 2001;134:963–7.

57. Lo CM, Liu CL, Chan SC, et al. A randomized, controlled trial of postoperative adjuvant interferon therapy after resection of hepatocellular carcinoma. Ann Surg 2007;245:831–42.

58. Belli G, Fantini C, D'Agostino A, et al. Laparoscopic versus open liver resection for hepatocellular carcinoma in patients with histologically proven cirrhosis: short- and middle-term results. Surg Endosc 2007;21:2004–11.

59. Mazzaferro V, Regalia E, Doci R, et al. Liver transplantation for the treatment of small hepatocellular carcinomas in patients with cirrhosis. N Engl J Med 1996; 334:693–9.

60. Yao FY, Kinkhabwala M, LaBerge JM, et al. The impact of pre-operative loco-regional therapy on outcome after liver transplantation for hepatocellular carcinoma. Am J Transplant 2005;5:795–804.

61. Onaca N, Davis GL, Goldstein RM, et al. Expanded criteria for liver transplantation in patients with hepatocellular carcinoma: a report from the International Registry of Hepatic Tumors in Liver Transplantation. Liver Transpl 2007;13:391–9.

62. Schwartz M. Liver transplantation for hepatocellular carcinoma. Gastroenterology 2004;127:S268–76.

63. Freeman RB Jr, Steffick DE, Guidinger MK, et al. Liver and intestine transplantation in the United States, 1997–2006. Am J Transplant 2008;8:958–76.

64. Yao FY, Hirose R, LaBerge JM, et al. A prospective study on downstaging of hepatocellular carcinoma prior to liver transplantation. Liver Transpl 2005;11: 1505–14.

65. Shetty K, Timmins K, Brensinger C, et al. Liver transplantation for hepatocellular carcinoma validation of present selection criteria in predicting outcome. Liver Transpl 2004;10:911–8.

66. Del Gaudio M, Grazi GL, Principe A, et al. Influence of prognostic factors on the outcome of liver transplantation for hepatocellular carcinoma on cirrhosis: a univariate and multivariate analysis. Hepatogastroenterology 2004;51:510–4.

67. Poon RT, Fan ST, Lo CM, et al. Difference in tumor invasiveness in cirrhotic patients with hepatocellular carcinoma fulfilling the Milan criteria treated by resection and transplantation: impact on long-term survival. Ann Surg 2007;245:51–8.

68. Galandi D, Antes G. Radiofrequency thermal ablation versus other interventions for hepatocellular carcinoma. Cochrane Database Syst Rev 2004;(2):CD003046.

69. Shiina S, Teratani T, Obi S, et al. A randomized controlled trial of radiofrequency ablation with ethanol injection for small hepatocellular carcinoma. Gastroenterology 2005;129:122–30.

70. Lin SM, Lin CJ, Lin CC, et al. Radiofrequency ablation improves prognosis compared with ethanol injection for hepatocellular carcinoma ≤4 cm. Gastroenterology 2004;127:1714–23.

71. Zhou XD, Tang ZY. Cryotherapy for primary liver cancer. Semin Surg Oncol 1998; 14:171–4.

72. Littlewood K. Anesthetic considerations for hepatic cryotherapy. Semin Surg Oncol 1998;14:116–21.

73. Hasegawa K, Makuuchi M, Takayama T, et al. Surgical resection vs. percutaneous ablation for hepatocellular carcinoma: a preliminary report of the Japanese nationwide survey. J Hepatol 2008;49:589–94.

74. Llovet JM, Bruix J. Systematic review of randomized trials for unresectable hepatocellular carcinoma: chemoembolization improves survival. Hepatology 2003;37:429–42.

75. Llovet JM, Real MI, Montana X, et al. Arterial embolisation or chemoembolisation versus symptomatic treatment in patients with unresectable hepatocellular carcinoma: a randomised controlled trial. Lancet 2002;359:1734–9.

76. Lo CM, Ngan H, Tso WK, et al. Randomized controlled trial of transarterial lipiodol chemoembolization for unresectable hepatocellular carcinoma. Hepatology 2002;35:1164–71.

77. Kulik LM, Carr BI, Mulcahy MF, et al. Safety and efficacy of 90Y radiotherapy for hepatocellular carcinoma with and without portal vein thrombosis. Hepatology 2008;47:71–81.

78. Bush DA, Hillebrand DJ, Slater JM, et al. High-dose proton beam radiotherapy of hepatocellular carcinoma: preliminary results of a phase II trial. Gastroenterology 2004;127:S189–93.

79. Varela M, Real MI, Burrel M, et al. Chemoembolization of hepatocellular carcinoma with drug eluting beads: efficacy and doxorubicin pharmacokinetics. J Hepatol 2007;46:474–81.

80. Llovet JM, Bruix J. Novel advancements in the management of hepatocellular carcinoma in 2008. J Hepatol 2008;48(Suppl 1):S20–37.

81. Llovet JM, Ricci S, Mazzaferro V, et al. Sorafenib in advanced hepatocellular carcinoma. N Engl J Med 2008;359:378–90.

Nonalcoholic Fatty Liver Disease: A Practical Approach to Evaluation and Management

Nila Rafiq, MD, Zobair M. Younossi, MD, MPH*

KEYWORDS

- Non-alcoholic fatty liver disease • Non-alcoholic steatohepatitis
- Obesity • Metabolic syndrome

Nonalcoholic fatty liver disease (NAFLD) is among the most common causes of chronic liver disease worldwide.[1] NAFLD encompasses a wide spectrum of clinicopathologic conditions, including simple steatosis and nonalcoholic steatohepatitis (NASH). Within the spectrum of NAFLD, only NASH has been convincingly shown to have a progressive course, potentially leading to cirrhosis, hepatocellular carcinoma, or liver failure. Most patients with NAFLD have risk factors, such as insulin resistance, obesity, or other components of the metabolic syndrome. NAFLD is now recognized as the hepatic manifestation of the metabolic syndrome. According to the Adult Treatment Panel III, metabolic syndrome encompasses 3 of the following components: the presence of visceral obesity (waist circumference of more than 40 inches in males and more than 35 inches in females), hypertension (HTN) with a blood pressure greater than 130/85 mm Hg, fasting blood glucose greater than 100 mg/dL, elevated triglycerides of 150 or greater, and a low high-density lipoprotein (HDL) of less than 40 in males and 50 in females. Population studies show higher liver-related mortality and cardiac mortality in patients with NAFLD.[2]

During the past few decades, NAFLD has continued to rise among adults, adolescents, and children, potentially increasing its mortality, morbidity, and economic impact. Many patients with NAFLD and NASH remain undiagnosed, and even after diagnosis of NAFLD, many health care practitioners mistakenly consider it benign.

EPIDEMIOLOGY

Published data are limited, but we know that NAFLD occurs among all ethnicities, genders, and all age groups, including children and adolescents. The true incidence

Center for Liver Diseases at Inova Fairfax Hospital, 3300 Gallows Road, Falls Church, VA 22042, USA
* Corresponding author.
E-mail address: zobair.younossi@inova.org (Z.M. Younossi).

Clin Liver Dis 13 (2009) 249–266
doi:10.1016/j.cld.2009.02.009
1089-3261/09/$ – see front matter © 2009 Elsevier Inc. All rights reserved.

liver.theclinics.com

and prevalence of NAFLD and NASH are unknown; however, studies have reported that approximately 25% to 30% of the US population is affected with NAFLD. NASH, the progressive form of NAFLD, has an estimated prevalence of 3% to 5%, and an estimated 9% to 15% of patients with NASH potentially progress to cirrhosis. The rise in NAFLD has paralleled increases in obesity and diabetes.[3] The World Health Organization has estimated that 1 billion people are overweight and another 300 million people are obese.[4] Furthermore, 47 million people in the United States are estimated to have metabolic syndrome, 80% of whom may have NAFLD.[5,6] Prevalence of NAFLD in morbidly obese is 93% and in type 2 diabetics is about 62%.[3]

The National Health and Nutrition Examination Survey (NHANES) has revealed that NAFLD occurs earlier in men around the fourth decade compared with women who present in the sixth decade. This prevalence rate increases with age. Cryptogenic liver enzyme elevation (presumed NAFLD) seems to be greatest among Mexican Americans in comparison with non-Hispanic or African Americans. Hispanics have a greater prevalence of NAFLD in comparison with non-Hispanic whites or non-Hispanic African Americans.[7–10]

Pediatric Nonalcoholic Fatty Liver Disease

Childhood obesity has also become a global epidemic.[11,12] According to NHANES (2003–2004), 17.1% of children and adolescents 2 to 19 years of age were considered to be overweight,[13] which has been defined as at or more than the 95th percentile of the sex-specific body mass index (BMI) for age growth charts. Most of this pediatric population will be overweight or obese as adults, and NAFLD is common in overweight or obese children. The diagnosis, treatment, and prevention of NAFLD have not been clearly defined in the pediatric population, as it is usually asymptomatic. It does not predominate in females in this population, and aminotransferases and triglycerides may be mildly elevated. NAFLD is more commonly recognized in children with metabolic syndrome due to childhood cancers, hypothalamic or pituitary dysfunction, changes in growth hormone secretion,[14–16] congenital forms of lipodystrophy,[17,18] Prader-Willi syndrome, and polycystic ovarian syndrome.[19,20] Rashid and Roberts[21] followed 36 patients with NAFLD from 4 to 16 years of age from 1985 through 1995. The majority of patients were overweight or frankly obese, with a male predominance. Liver biopsies were performed in 24 patients, and 71% showed fibrosis, and 1 patient had cirrhosis.[21] In a clinical series from San Diego, California, 43 children of various ethnicities were noted to have histologic NAFLD. Among this cohort, 75% had hyperinsulinemia as well as insulin resistance by the homeostasis model of insulin resistance.[22] Another study reported that children and adolescents with a family history of metabolic syndrome or fatty liver are at a greater risk for having NAFLD.[23]

NATURAL HISTORY

The natural history of NAFLD has become better defined, as understanding of the disease process has become more sophisticated, and longer follow-up data have become available. Evidence to date indicates that simple steatosis is generally nonprogressive, but a small percentage of patients with simple steatosis may progress to NASH with potential progression to cirrhosis. NASH is the potentially progressive form of NAFLD. NASH has been divided into primary and secondary types. As noted previously, "primary" NASH is associated with obesity-related conditions and insulin resistance, whereas "secondary" NASH reflects medication use and other nonmetabolic causes.

Evidence for the progressive nature of NASH comes from a variety of studies.[24–27] One report described 132 patients with biopsy-proven NAFLD who had a mean follow-up time of 8.17 years, with the longest follow-up being 18 years. Liver-related mortality was approximately 11.7% in NASH but only 1.7% in non-NASH patients (simple steatosis and simple steatosis with inflammation).[24] Approximately 10 years later, the same cohort of NAFLD patients had a median follow-up of 18.5 years, the longest being 28.5 years. After a median follow-up of almost 2 decades, liver-related mortality had increased to 17.5% in NASH and 2.7% in non-NASH patients.[28] The 3 most frequent causes of death were cardiovascular malignancy, and hepatic-related deaths.[24,28] In contrast, in the general population, liver-related mortality is the 13th cause of death. Another long-term follow up study evaluated 129 biopsy-proven NAFLD patients with a mean follow-up of 13.7 years. Approximately 80% of these patients developed diabetes or insulin resistance. These investigators reported an increase in liver-related mortality only in the NASH cohort. The 3 most frequent causes of death were similar to those in the previous study: cardiovascular, malignancy, and liver-related deaths.[29]

Another study illustrating the progressive course of NASH reported sequential liver biopsies in 252 patients. About 31% had an increase in fibrosis, and 9% showed progression to cirrhosis.[3]

Further evidence to support the progressive nature of NASH comes from community-based data from Olmstead County, Minnesota, where 450 patients with NAFLD were followed from 1980 to 2000 for an average of 7.6 years. Survival was lower in the NAFLD cohort than that in the general population. The third leading cause of death was liver-related deaths. Higher mortality was associated with older age, impaired fasting glucose, and cirrhosis.[30]

Additional evidence supporting the progressive nature of NASH has come from population-based studies. A study based on NHANES III data linked to National Death Index mortality files reported on a total of 12,822 patients, consisting of 817 patients with NAFLD, 1,537 patients with other liver diseases, and the remaining with no liver disease. A total of 1,533 deaths occurred during 8.74 years; 80 patients were diagnosed with NAFLD, and 1,453 had no evidence of liver disease. Liver-related death was again the third most frequent cause of death after cardiovascular and malignancy deaths.[2]

Finally, evidence of the progressive nature of NASH comes from a study of cryptogenic cirrhosis and hepatocellular carcinoma. Patients with cryptogenic cirrhosis were similar to patients with NASH with regard to the prevalence of diabetes and obesity. Patients with cryptogenic cirrhosis were typically 10 years older than the NASH patients. Furthermore, many patients who had received a liver transplant for cryptogenic cirrhosis usually developed graft NAFLD/NASH post-transplantation.[31] Also, in a study of 105 patients with hepatocellular carcinoma, 29% (n = 30) had cryptogenic cirrhosis. Approximately 47% of these patients had clinical or histologic evidence of NAFLD.[32]

Together, these studies suggest that NASH is a serious liver disease with 10% to 15% of patients progressing to cirrhosis within a few decades.

CLINICAL AND HISTOLOGIC PREDICTORS OF NONALCOHOLIC STEATOHEPATITIS

Apart from histologic findings, there are no reliable criteria for predicting which NAFLD patients will progress to fibrosis or advanced liver disease. Specific histologic and clinical factors predicting a progressive course are currently being evaluated. In a study of NAFLD patients, a higher grade of fibrosis was independently associated with the presence of hepatocyte ballooning: Mallory bodies on biopsy as well as a higher aspartate aminotransferase (AST)/alanine aminotransferase (ALT) ratio.[33] Marchesini and colleagues[6] reported that the metabolic syndrome is independently associated with the presence of histologic NASH and fibrosis. Another study evaluating NAFLD patients found that compared with nondiabetics with NAFLD, those with diabetes had higher rates of cirrhosis, liver-related mortality, and overall mortality.[34] Angulo and colleagues[35] assessed 144 patients with NASH. Independent predictors of advanced fibrosis included age more than 45 years, AST/ALT more than 1, obesity, and the presence of diabetes. Morbidly obese patients with NAFLD who underwent bariatric surgery were evaluated by Dixon and colleagues[36]; independent predictors of NASH included insulin resistance, elevated ALT, and a history of systemic HTN.

NONALCOHOLIC FATTY LIVER DISEASE AND CARDIOVASCULAR DISEASE

As previously noted, NAFLD and cardiovascular disease, including coronary artery disease (CAD) and cerebrovascular disease, are the hepatic and cardiac manifestations of the metabolic syndrome. Long-term studies indicate that cardiovascular mortality is the commonest cause of death in NAFLD patients. In a study of 92 patients undergoing coronary angiography, approximately 71% had fatty liver on ultrasound (US). Furthermore, NAFLD independently increased the risk for CAD.[37] Targher and coworkers found that patients with NAFLD and type II diabetes had a higher prevalence of cardiovascular disease and increased cardiac mortality.[38] Although several mechanisms (endothelial dysfunction, increased arthrosclerosis, and so forth) have been implicated, further studies are required to understand the relationship between NAFLD and cardiovascular disease.

PATHOPHYSIOLOGY

Several mechanisms have been postulated to explain the pathogenesis of NASH. The "multiple hit" hypotheses is currently favored. The first "hit" is development of hepatic macrosteatosis as a result of increased lipolysis and free fatty acids. Postulated mechanisms leading to hepatic steatosis include increased lipogenesis, decreased lipid export, and a reduction of free fatty acid oxidation with insulin resistance leading to fatty acid dysregulation.

Several potential "second hits" include oxidative stress from reactive oxygen species in the mitochondria and cytochrome P450 enzymes. Other second hits include the presence of endotoxins, cytokines, adipokines, and environmental factors. Central obesity with visceral fat and white adipose deposition is a major source of adipokines and cytokines in NAFLD patients. Adipokines released from white adipose tissue include adiponectin (protective), leptin (pro-fibrotic), and resistin (mediator of IR). Others include visfatin, vaspin and apelin which are potentially involved in IR. The proinflammatory cytokines released from white adipose tissue include tumor necrosis factor alpha (TNF-α) and interleukin-6. Initial data support a role for adipokines and cytokines in the pathogenesis of NASH, but additional studies are needed to validate this relationship. For more detail regarding the pathogenesis of NAFLD, refer to the article by Edmison and McCullough.[39]

CLINICAL PRESENTATION

The majority of patients with NAFLD and NASH are asymptomatic with mild, incidental elevation of aminotransferases. No specific symptoms can distinguish NAFLD or

NASH from other types of liver disease. The diagnosis of NAFLD requires the exclusion of other specific etiologies of liver disease and excessive alcohol consumption. The majority of patients have 1 or more risk factors for metabolic syndrome, such as type 2 diabetes, obesity, HTN, or hyperlipidemia. When symptoms occur, the most common complaint is fatigue and occasionally right upper quadrant abdominal discomfort.

No specific findings on physical examination identify patients with NAFLD. However, the most common abnormality is the presence of central adiposity. Physical signs of metabolic syndrome and insulin resistance, such as acanthosis nigricans, may be observed to occur in younger patients. In addition, mild hepatomegaly may be noted in some patients with NAFLD.[1,40] If liver disease is advanced, cutaneous stigmata of cirrhosis may be present with features of portal HTN.

DIAGNOSIS

NAFLD should be suspected as a cause of asymptomatic elevation of aminotransferases as discussed elsewhere in this issue of *Clinics of Liver Disease*. However, it is important to remember that NAFLD can be present with normal or fluctuating AST and ALT. In general, ALT is higher than AST. Nevertheless, similar to other types of liver diseases, an AST/ALT ratio greater than 1 may indicate advanced fibrosis. The diagnosis of NAFLD is strongly suggested when metabolic syndrome is present and other specific etiologies for hepatic dysfunction have been excluded. Various tests for diagnosis and staging NASH are shown in **Fig. 1**.[41] The role of various diagnostic modalities in NAFLD is summarized next.

Radiologic Modalities

NAFLD is most commonly suggested by an asymptomatic elevation of liver enzymes or fatty infiltration apparent in imaging. Ultrasound (US) may show liver steatosis as a hyperechogenic image, that is, "bright liver." Radiologic techniques used to evaluate NAFLD include US, computed tomography, magnetic resonance imaging, and

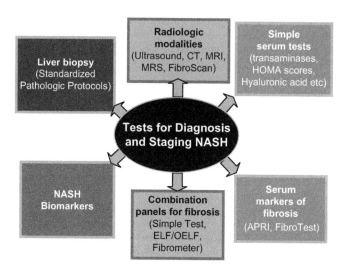

Fig. 1. Tests for diagnosis and staging of NASH. (*Modified from* Baranova A, Younossi ZM. The future is around the corner: non-invasive diagnosis of the progressive nonalcoholic steatohepatitis. Hepatology 2008;47(2):373–5; with permission.)

magnetic resonance spectroscopy (MRS). However, these radiologic modalities are accurate in detecting hepatic steatosis only when there is moderate to severe steatosis. On the other hand, sensitivity is highly variable with mild degrees of steatosis and in patients who are morbidly obese. Although these modalities can detect hepatic steatosis, none is able to distinguish simple steatosis from NASH or determine the stage of hepatic fibrosis.[42]

A noninvasive radiologic technique currently under evaluation is MRS. This technique measures hepatic triglycerides quantitatively. It is noninvasive, safe, and reproducible but requires further testing to determine its effectiveness for stage of fibrosis in NAFLD.[43]

Transient elastography (Fibroscan) is currently being evaluated for stage of fibrosis in NAFLD. This noninvasive test for the assessment of liver fibrosis measures the hepatic stiffness. In a study of 711 patients with chronic liver disease, including chronic hepatitis B, C, and NASH, liver stiffness correlated with the extent of liver fibrosis.[44] Fibroscan's role in obese NAFLD patients remains to be established.[45]

Dual energy X-ray absorptiometry evaluates body fat distribution. This technique can also be used to monitor various treatments and their effect on NAFLD and fat distribution.[46] Its role in NAFLD remains experimental.

In summary, imaging is frequently used in the evaluation of patients with NAFLD, but current routine radiologic modalities have limited value in this setting. Newer radiologic modalities represent a tremendous opportunity in NAFLD diagnostics.

Histology

As previously noted, histologic criteria for the diagnosis of NAFLD require 5% to 10% hepatic steatosis (predominantly macrovesicular) with or without other pathologic features. Several approaches have attempted to better define and describe the types of NAFLD. In the late 1990s, Younossi and colleagues[47] described 4 types of NAFLD (types 1–4) and assessed the inter- and intraobserver variability. These pathologic criteria were used to obtain clinical and pathologic data evaluating a cohort of NAFLD patients. All liver biopsies were read in a standardized approach by 1 hepatopathologist with 4 histologic criteria: type 1, simple steatosis alone; type 2, simple steatosis plus lobular inflammation; type 3, steatosis and ballooning degeneration; and type 4, as in type 3 plus either Mallory's hyaline or fibrosis. Long-term outcomes revealed that types 1 and 2 NAFLD followed a nonprogressive course, in contrast to types 3 and 4 NAFLD, which had a progressive course.[24]

Brunt and coworkers subsequently developed a scoring system incorporating NAFLD grade and staging. Stage 1 NASH was described as steatosis in zone 3, occasional ballooning, and intra-acinar inflammation with pericellular fibrosis. Stage 2 was similar to stage 1 but with the presence of sinusoidal and periportal fibrosis. Stage 3 presented with bridging fibrosis between zones 3 and 1, and stage 4 indicated cirrhosis.[48]

Finally, the NASH Clinical Research Network has created a histologic scoring system for diagnosis of NAFLD. The NAFLD Activity Score (NAS) evaluated 3 pathologic features: macrosteatosis in zone 3, inflammation, and hepatocyte ballooning. Additional features for strengthening the diagnosis of NASH include Mallory's hyaline, perisinusoidal fibrosis, portal inflammation, acidophilic bodies, glycogenated nuclei, periodic acid stain after diastase Kupffer cells and lipogranulomas. Histologic activity is graded 0 to 8 and fibrosis, 0 to 4. NASH is confirmed with a score of 5 or greater.[49] It is important to remember that the NAS scoring system was developed for clinical trials of NASH and has not been used extensively in clinical practice to establish the diagnosis of NASH.

Histologic features of NASH differ in children and adults. Children usually present with a mononuclear inflammatory infiltrate that is periportal rather than perivenular. Mallory bodies are rarely present in pediatric NAFLD, and fibrosis has a periportal rather than pericellular distribution.[21,50,51]

Additionally, the pathologic features of NASH in morbidly obese patients may be different, showing changes in the portal area rather than central areas of a liver biopsy.

Another important issue related to liver biopsy is the risk, cost, and sampling error related to liver biopsy in NAFLD. Despite these shortcomings, liver biopsy remains the "imperfect" gold standard for diagnosis of NASH.

Nonalcoholic Fatty Liver Disease Biomarkers

Many biomarkers are being evaluated for the diagnosis of NASH. The most useful biomarkers are noninvasive, simple, accurate, and inexpensive.[41] Three types of biomarkers are under assessment for clinical use: NASH diagnostic biomarkers that can replace the need for a liver biopsy, biomarkers assessing hepatic steatosis, and biomarkers to stage hepatic fibrosis in NASH.

As noted previously, a proinflammatory state and oxidative stress play important roles in the pathogenesis of NAFLD, as does apoptosis.[3,52–54] Cytokeratin 18 (CK-18) and caspase-cleaved CK-18 are elevated in patients with NASH. Furthermore, CK-18 fragments seem to be able to independently predict NASH on multivariate analysis with an area under the curve (AUC) of 0.93. The diagnosis of NASH had a specificity of 94% and sensitivity of 90.5%.[52,53]

Another study used a combination of biomarkers including cleaved CK-18, M30 and M65 antigen, adiponectin, and resistin. The authors report an AUC of 0.908 with a sensitivity of 95.45% and sensitivity of 70.21% for diagnosis of NASH.[54] Large-scale external validation is still pending.

A second type of biomarker may assess the extent of hepatic steatosis. The Fatty Liver Index (FLI) was created by Bedogni and colleagues[55] to determine the presence of hepatic steatosis. The model includes 4 predictors: triglycerides, BMI, gamma-glutamyl transpeptidase (GGT), and waist circumference. Hepatic steatosis was excluded if the FLI less than 30 and included if it is more than 60. The diagnosis of fatty liver was also made by abdominal US.

A third type of biomarker is designed to estimate hepatic fibrosis. FibroTest (Fibro-Sure) and ActiTest are both noninvasive blood tests that provide an alternative to liver biopsy. Initially they were developed for viral hepatitis but are now being tested for NAFLD. They measure both necroinflammatory activity and fibrosis with 5 markers: α2-macroglobulin, apolipoprotein A1, haptoglobulin, total bilirubin, and GGT corrected for age and gender. The ActiTest includes the FibroTest plus ALT. However, these tests are not accurate in patients with Gilbert's syndrome, cholestasis, and acute inflammation.[56]

Two other tests have been developed to detect the presence of steatosis or NASH. The SteatoTest is a panel of noninvasive biomarkers to predict steatosis. It uses the FibroTest-ActiTest plus BMI, glucose, triglycerides, and cholesterol adjusted to age and gender.[57] The NashTest varies slightly in that it attempts to distinguish simple steatosis from NASH.[58]

The AST/platelets ratio index test is a predictive panel for detection of fibrosis, which consists of 2 parameters incorporating ALT/platelets ratio index.[59] The Fibrometer is a noninvasive marker of fibrosis including platelet count, prothrombin index, AST, α2-macroglobulin, hyaluronate, urea, and age.[60]

Angulo and colleagues[61] have developed a scoring system to distinguish NAFLD patients with and without fibrosis. It consists of 6 variables including age, BMI, hyperglycemia, platelet count, albumin, and AST/ALT ratio. The estimation and valida-tion groups had receiver operating characteristic curves of 0.88 and 0.82. The scoring system was able to accurately identify patients at risk for fibrosis.

The Original European Liver Fibrosis (OELF) panel determines the extent of hepatic fibrosis by evaluating age, hyaluronic acid, amino-terminal propeptide of type III collagen, and tissue inhibitor of matrix metalloproteinase.[62] ELF is the simplified version of OELF, which does not include age and has been shown to predict fibrosis in NAFLD patients.[63] Although increasingly better tests are being developed, the current generation of biomarkers for NASH or fibrosis (in patients with NASH) are not fully validated for clinical use.

TREATMENT OF NONALCOHOLIC FATTY LIVER DISEASE

There is no approved therapy for NAFLD. Currently, patients with NAFLD are advised to address risk factors for metabolic syndrome, which include insulin resistance, systemic HTN, and hypercholesteremia and obesity.

Interventions are currently targeted to patients with NASH rather than simple stea-tosis because of its potential to progress to cirrhosis. A suggested algorithm for the management of NAFLD is shown in **Fig. 2**.

Lifestyle Changes

The initially attempted management of NAFLD includes weight reduction through life-style modifications with diet and exercise. No randomized clinical trials have evaluated the effects of weight loss for treatment of NAFLD. However, weight loss has been shown to decrease adipose tissue, which leads to reduced insulin resistance. Specif-ically, aerobic exercise may prevent the development of steatosis. Insulin sensitivity is increased through peripheral lipolysis, inhibiting lipid synthesis and enabling fatty acid oxidation.[64] A target loss of 10% of the baseline weight should be the initial goal for a BMI greater than 25; this reduces aminotransferase levels and diminishes hepato-megaly.[65] Weight loss through diet and exercise should be gradual. Rapid weight loss exceeding 1.6 kg/wk has the potential to worsen steatohepatitis and cause gallstones.[66] Palmer and Schaffner[65] placed 39 patients on very low-calorie diet (600–800 kcal/d) combined with exercise. The patients who lost greater than 10% of their ideal body weight had reduced aminotransferases. A study evaluating 25 Japanese patients with NAFLD included 15 patients who were placed on a restricted diet and exercise for 3 months. These patients had improvements in BMI, aminotrans-ferases, total cholesterol, and decreased serum glucose compared with those of the control group. Steatosis improved on liver biopsy, but there was no reduction in inflammation or fibrosis.[67]

Diet

Because the majority of patients have difficulty losing and maintaining weight loss, it is recommended that in addition to exercise, patients be counseled on nutrition and diet. Insulin resistance has been shown to worsen with saturated fat consump-tion[68–70] but may improve with a high-fiber diet.[71,72] Two studies have suggested that a calorie-restricted diet with or without exercise may induce biochemical improvement in overweight and obese patients suspected to have NAFLD.[65,67,73] Although these diets may assist in losing weight, their effects on NAFLD have not been carefully examined.

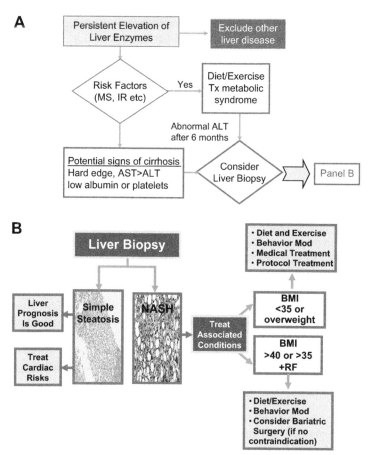

Fig. 2. Management algorithm for NAFLD. (*A*) Elevation of Liver Enzyme evaluation. (*B*) Liver Biopsy evaluation.

Antiobesity Medications

Two medications have been approved for weight loss: orlistat and sibutramine. Orlistat is an enteric lipase inhibitor that blocks the absorption of long-chain fatty acids and cholesterol. In a study with biopsy-proven NASH, orlistat decreased weight by 10.3 kg. There was also significant biochemical improvement and a reduction in BMI.[74] Sibutramine stimulates weight loss by inhibiting serotonin and norepinephrine reuptake and increasing satiety. Sabuncu and colleagues[75] compared orlistat to sibutramine in 25 patients. Six months of therapy resulted in a reduction of insulin resistance, weight loss, improved aminotransferases, and sonographic evidence of hepatic steatosis. Rimonabant, another antiobesity medication, is an antagonist of the cannabinoid receptor type 1 (CB1). Rimonabant administered to obese fa/fa obese rats resulted in the disappearance of steatosis and a reduction in liver enzymes, triglycerides, and fatty acids.[76] Although these antiobesity medications may be effective for weight reduction, randomized clinical trials are needed to determine their safety efficacy in NAFLD. In fact, recent data suggesting a potential association between CB1 antagonists and depression has raised concerns about the long term use of these drugs in NAFLD.

Bariatric Surgery

Treatment for NASH may include bariatric surgery categorized as restrictive, malabsorptive, or mixed restrictive-malabsorptive types. Surgery is recommended for patients with a BMI greater than 40 or a BMI greater than 35 with comorbid conditions. Laparoscopic adjustable gastric banding (LAGB) and vertical banded gastroplasty are restrictive procedures that decrease the stomach size. Roux-en-Y gastric bypass and duodenal switch remove a great portion of the small intestine, causing malabsorption of fats and nutrients. Losing weight decreases white adipose tissue, hepatic steatosis, improves insulin sensitivity, and also decreases inflammatory markers.[77] A study of patients undergoing LAGB showed a 34 ± 17 kg weight loss with improved metabolic syndrome. In addition, NASH resolved in 82% of patients.[78] Other beneficial effects include improvements in sleep apnea, depression, infertility, and quality of life.[78] A Swedish Obese Study Group proposed a better long-term outcome of cardiovascular risk factors, such as diabetes, hypertriglyceridemia, and HTN, in patients who had undergone bariatric surgery.[79] Maggard and colleagues[80] in a meta-analysis of 147 studies reported that weight loss and obesity-related conditions were more successful in patients undergoing bariatric surgery in comparison with medical treatment. Many other studies have demonstrated similar results.

Pharmacologic Treatment of Insulin Resistance

As previously noted, insulin resistance is an important component in the pathophysiology of NASH. Features of the metabolic syndrome and insulin resistance are present in more than 80% of patients with NASH. Pharmacologic therapy is aimed at treating insulin resistance. Drugs currently under investigation for insulin resistance include metformin and thiazolidinediones.

Biguanide

Metformin is a biguanide that improves insulin resistance by decreasing the production of hepatic glucose and increasing the uptake of peripheral glucose by skeletal muscle and fatty acid oxidation. In addition, metformin can improve TNF-α-induced insulin resistance. Small trials have shown biochemical and histologic improvement in NASH with no associated weight gain. Nondiabetic patients in an open-label study were placed on metformin 2 gm daily, a weight reducing diet, or vitamin E 800 IU. The metformin group had a fall in ALT and improved steatosis, inflammation, and fibrosis in comparison with vitamin E.[81] A study using metformin 2 gm daily showed biochemical improvement after 3 months but no significant difference at month 12.[82]

Thiazolidinediones

Thiazolidinediones are oral antidiabetic medications that are currently being tested for treatment of NASH. They bind to peroxisome proliferator-activated receptor gamma (PPAR-γ) and decrease insulin resistance by various mechanisms. They stimulate free fatty acid oxidation, increase adiponectin expression, and have been shown in obese rats to decrease triglycerides and TNF-α.[83] Furthermore, a study of diabetic patients showed that troglitazone reduced leptin levels.[84]

A number of clinical trials have assessed the efficacy of thiazolidinediones in patients with NASH. Neuschwander-Tetri and colleagues[85] treated 30 patients with biopsy-proven NASH using 4 mg of rosiglitazone and showed an improvement in insulin resistance, aminotransferases, and liver histology after 48 weeks of treatment. However, after discontinuing rosiglitazone, the improvement in liver enzymes reversed in association with weight gain. Another study testing rosiglitazone in patients with NASH revealed improved steatosis and insulin sensitivity and reduced aminotransferases.[86] However, weight gain was a prominent side effect. After 1 year of treatment, only half the patients showed histologic improvement. Furthermore, recent studies have shown that thiazolidinediones increase cardiovascular risks,[87] osteoporosis,[88] and weight gain. Similar efficacey data of Pioglitazon has been shown in patients with NASH.[89] These potential side effects must be considered when considering the long term use of these regimens for patients with NASH.

Lipid-Lowering Agents

Elevated triglycerides and low HDL are components of the metabolic syndrome associated with NAFLD. Several studies have investigated the effect of hyperlipidemia treatment on NAFLD. Hydroxymethylglutaryl-CoA reductase inhibitors are known to potentially cause hepatotoxicity; 2 studies show that it does in fact reduce ALT.[90,91] Pravastatin 20 mg daily was used to treat hyperlipidemia for 6 months; liver enzymes normalized and hepatic inflammation decreased.[92] Another study showed improvement in the lipid profile as well as aminotransferases with use of atorvastatin.[93] It has recently been shown that liver fibrosis did not progress in patients on statins for 10.3 to 16.3 years.[94]

Gemfibrozil, a fibric acid derivative, is another lipid-lowering agent; patients treated with 600 mg daily for 4 weeks showed biochemical improvement.[95] In animal models, clofibrate revealed a reduction in hepatic triglycerides. Nevertheless, an open-label trial showed no biochemical or histologic improvement.[96]

Antioxidants

Oxidative stress plays a major role in the multihit hypothesis of NAFLD. Several studies have evaluated the effects of antioxidants in patients with NAFLD. Two trials suggested that vitamin E is beneficial,[97,98] but 2 others showed that it was ineffective.[99,100] A randomized study comparing vitamin E and vitamin C to placebo for 6 months showed no improvement in aminotransferases and histology.[101]

Betaine is a metabolite of choline and increases S-adenosylmethionin levels, which has been shown to be hepatoprotective. A small study of 10 patients with NASH treated with betaine showed a reduction in AST, ALT, steatosis, inflammation, and fibrosis after 1 year.[102] Apparently, a subsequent RCT of this agent did not show significant efficacy.

Ursodeoxycholic Acid

The hepatoprotective effects of ursodeoxycholic acid (UDCA) are currently under investigation as potential treatment for NAFLD. A small study of 24 patients with NASH treated with UDCA at 13 to 15 mg/d showed a reduction in steatosis and serum liver enzyme levels after 2 years of treatment.[96] Lindor and colleagues[103] conducted a randomized, double-blind, controlled trial comparing UDCA and placebo in 166 patients with NASH. Treatment was well tolerated but, unfortunately, there was no biochemical or histologic improvement.

Angiotensin-Converting Enzyme Inhibitor/Angiotensin Receptor Blocker

Several studies have attempted treatment of the metabolic syndrome. Angiotensin-converting enzyme inhibitors (ACE-Is) and angiotensin receptor blockers (ARBs) may prevent type 2 diabetes in patients with HTN or congestive heart failure. ACE-Is suppress the renin angiotensin system. ARBs, irbesartan, and telmisartan, are thought to activate PPAR-γ and decrease insulin resistance. A small study treating 7 patients with NASH and HTN with losartan for 48 weeks reported a reduction in aminotransferases, serum markers of fibrosis, and histologic improvement.[104]

Other Novel Agents

Pentoxifylline has also been used to treat NAFLD. It functions by inhibiting TNF-α, which is implicated in the multihit hypothesis of NASH. A few small studies have shown that pentoxifylline may improve aminotransferases in patients with NASH.[105,106]

Because some studies have suggested an overgrowth of intestinal bacteria in NASH, probiotics are under investigation for NASH treatment. Researchers have shown improved ALT and other markers of lipid peroxidation with the use of probiotic VSL#3 in NAFLD patients.[107]

An insulin secretagogue, nateglinide, improves biochemical and histologic parameters in diabetic patients with NASH.[108] However, large randomized trials are required to determine the effectiveness of these treatments in patients with NASH.

SUMMARY

NAFLD is a leading cause of chronic liver disease worldwide. NASH, the progressive form of NAFLD, may progress to cirrhosis, liver failure, or hepatocellular carcinoma. Its prevalence and the overall and liver-related mortality are expected to increase with the increased rates of obesity and type 2 diabetes. Therefore, it is important to diagnose NAFLD and identify patients with NASH. However, no single diagnostic or noninvasive test can reliably detect NASH besides liver biopsy. Treatment of NAFLD will require effective preventive and therapeutic modalities. Current therapies for NAFLD include weight loss through lifestyle modifications and treatment for insulin resistance and the other components of metabolic syndrome. However, the effectiveness of these therapies needs further evaluation in randomized, double-blind, controlled trials.

REFERENCES

1. Ludwig J, Viggiano TR, McGill DB, et al. Nonalcoholic steatohepatitis: Mayo Clinic experiences with a hitherto unnamed disease. Mayo Clin Proc 1980;55: 434–8.
2. Ong JP, Pitts A, Younossi ZM, et al. Increased overall mortality and liver-related mortality in non-alcoholic fatty liver disease. J Hepatol 2008;49(4):608–12.
3. Ong JP, Younossi ZM. Approach to the diagnosis and treatment of nonalcoholic fatty liver disease. Clin Liver Dis 2005;9(4):617–34.
4. Obesity and Overweight. World Health Organization Web site. Available at: http://www.who.int/dietphysicalactivity/publications/facts/obesity/en/. Accessed December 10, 2007.
5. Ford ES, Giles WH, Dietz WH. Prevalence of the metabolic syndrome among US adults: findings from the Third National Health and Nutrition Examination Survey. JAMA 2002;287:356–9.
6. Marchesini G, Bugianesi E, Forlani G, et al. Nonalcoholic fatty liver, steatohepatitis, and the metabolic syndrome. Hepatology 2003;37(4):917–23.
7. Clark JM, Brancati FL, Diehl AM. The prevalence and etiology of elevated aminotransferase levels in the United States. AM J Gastroenterol 2003;98(5): 960–7.
8. McCullough AJ. The epidemiology and risk factors of NASH. In: Farrell GC, George J, Hall P, editors. Fatty liver disease: NASH and related disorders. Oxford (UK): Blackwell Publishing; 2005. p. 23–7.
9. Weston SR, Leyden W, Murphy R, et al. Racial and ethnic distribution of nonalcoholic fatty liver in persons with newly diagnosed chronic liver disease. Hepatology 2005;41(2):372–9.

10. Caldwell SH, Harris DM, Patrie JT, et al. Is NASH underdiagnosed among African Americans? Am J Gastroenterol 2002;97(6):1496–500.
11. Lobstein T, Baur L, Uauy R. Obesity in children and young people: a crisis in public health. Obes Rev 2004;5(Suppl 1):4–104.
12. Ogden CI, Carroll MD, Curtin LR, et al. Prevalence of overweight and obesity in the United States, 1999–2004. JAMA 2006;295(13):1549–55.
13. Prevalence of Overweight Among Children and Adolescents: United States, 2003–2004. National Center for Health Statistics Web site. Available at: http://www.cdc.gov/nchs/products/pubs/pubd/hestats/overweight/overwght_child_03.htm. Accessed August 26, 2008.
14. Talvensaari KK, Lanning M, Tapanainen P, et al. Long-term survivors of childhood cancer have an increased risk of manifesting the metabolic syndrome. J Clin Endocrinol Metab 1996;81(8):3051–5.
15. Adams LA, Feldstein A, Lindor KD, et al. Nonalcoholic fatty liver disease among patients with hypothalamic and pituitary dysfunction. Hepatology 2004;39(4):909–14.
16. Srinivasan S, Ogle GD, Garnett SP, et al. Features of the metabolic syndrome after childhood craniophayngioma. J Clin Endocrinol Metab 2004;89(1):81–6.
17. Powell EE, Searle J, Mortimer R. Steatohepatitis associated with limb lipodystrophy. Gastroenterology 1989;97(4):1022–4.
18. Cauble MS, Gilroy R, Sorrell MF, et al. Lipoatrophic diabetes and end-stage liver disease secondary to nonalcoholic steatohepatitis with recurrence after liver transplantation. Transplantation 2001;71(7):892–5.
19. Yigit S, Estrada E, Bucci K, et al. Diabetic ketoacidosis secondary to growth hormone treatment in a boy with Prader-Willi syndrome and steatohepatitis. J Pediatr Endocrinol Metab 2004;17(3):361–4.
20. Setji TL, Holland ND, Sanders LL, et al. Nonalcoholic steatohepatitis and nonalcoholic fatty liver disease in young women with polycystic ovary syndrome. J Clin Endorinol Metab 2006;91(5):1741–7.
21. Rashid M, Roberts EA. Nonalcoholic steatohepatitis in children. J Pediatr Gastroenterol Nutr 2000;30(1):48–53.
22. Schwimmer JB, Deutsch R, Rauch JB, et al. Obesity, insulin resistance, and other clinicopathological correlates of pediatric nonalcoholic fatty liver disease. J Pediatr 2003;143(4):500–5.
23. Willner IR, Waters B, Patil SR, et al. Ninety patients with nonalcoholic steatohepatitis: insulin resistance, familial tendency, and severity of disease. Am J Gastroenterol 2001;96(10):2957–61.
24. Matteoni CA, Younossi ZM, Gramlich T, et al. Nonalcoholic fatty liver disease: a spectrum of clinical and pathological severity. Gastroenterology 1999;116:1413–9.
25. Teli MR, James OFW, Burt AD, et al. The natural history of nonalcoholic fatty liver. A follow-up study. Hepatology 1995;22:1714–9.
26. Dam-Larsen S, Franzmann M, Anderson IB, et al. Long term prognosis of fatty liver disease and death. Gut 2004;53:750–5.
27. Powell EE, Cooksley WG, Hanson R, et al. The natural history of nonalcoholic steatohepatitis: a follow-up study of forty-two patients for up to 21 years. Hepatology 1990;11:74–80.
28. Rafiq N, Bai C, Younossi ZM, et al. Long term follow-up of patients with nonalcoholic fatty liver. Clin Gastroenterol Hepatol 2009;7(2):234–8.
29. Ekstedt M, Franzen LE, Mathiesen UL, et al. Long-term follow-up of patients with NAFLD and elevated liver enzymes. Hepatology 2006;44(4):865–73.

30. Adams LA, Lymp JF, St. Sauver J, et al. The natural history of nonalcoholic fatty liver disease: a population-based cohort study. Gastroenterology 2005;129: 113–21.

31. Caldwell SH, Oelsner DH, Iezzoni JC, et al. Cryptogenic cirrhosis: clinical characterization and risk factors for underlying disease. Hepatology 1999;29(3): 664–9.

32. Marrero JA, Fontana RJ, Su GL, et al. NAFLD may be a common underlying liver disease in patients with hepatocellular carcinoma in the United States. Hepatology 2002;36(6):1349–54.

33. Gramlich T, Kleiner DE, McCullogh AJ, et al. Pathologic features associated with fibrosis in nonalcoholic fatty liver disease. Hum Pathol 2004;35:196–9.

34. Younossi ZM, Gramlich T, Matteoni CA, et al. Nonalcoholic fatty liver disease in patients with type 2 diabetes. Clin Gastroenterol Hepatol 2004;2(3):262–5.

35. Angulo P, Keach JC, Batts KP, et al. Independent predictors of liver fibrosis in patients with nonalcoholic steatohepatitis. Hepatology 1999;30:1356–62.

36. Dixon JB, Bhathal PS, O'Brien PE. Nonalcoholic fatty liver disease: predictors of nonalcoholic steatohepatitis and liver fibrosis in the severely obese. Gastroenterology 2001;121:91–100.

37. Arslan U, Türkoğlu S, Balcioğlu S, et al. Association between nonalcoholic fatty liver disease and coronary artery disease. Coron Artery Dis 2007;18(6):433–6.

38. Targher G, Bertolini L, Padovani R, et al. Increased prevalence of cardiovascular disease in Type 2 diabetic patients with non-alcoholic fatty liver disease. Diabet Med 2006;23(4):403–9.

39. Edmison J, McCullough AJ. Pathogenesis of non-alchoholic steatohepatitis: human data. Clin Liver Dis 2007;11(1):75–104.

40. Bacon BR, Farahvash MJ, Janney CG, et al. Nonalcoholic steatohepatitis: an expanded clinical entity. Gastroenterology 1994;107:1103–9.

41. Baranova A, Younossi ZM. The future is around the corner: noninvasive diagnosis of progressive nonalcoholic steatohepatitis. Hepatology 2008;47(2): 373–5.

42. Saadeh S, Younossi ZM, Remer EM, et al. The utility of radiological imaging in nonalcoholic fatty liver disease. Gastroenterology 2002;123:745–50.

43. Szczepaniak LS, Nurenberg P, Leonard D, et al. Magnetic resonance spectroscopy to measure hepatic triglyceride content: prevalence of hepatic steatosis in the general population. Am J Physiol Endocrinol Metab 2005;288:E462–8.

44. Foucher J, Chanteloup E, Vergniol J, et al. Diagnosis of cirrhosis by transient elastography (Fibroscan): a prospective study. Gut 2006;55:403–8.

45. Ziol M, Handra-Luca A, Kettaneh A, et al. Noninvasive assessment of liver fibrosis by measurement of liver stiffness in patients with chronic hepatitis C. Hepatology 2005;41:48–54.

46. Promrat K, Lutchman G, Uwaifo GI, et al. A pilot study of pioglitazone treatment for nonalcoholic steatohepatitis. Hepatology 2004;39:188–96.

47. Younossi ZM, Gramlich T, Liu YC, et al. Nonalcoholic fatty liver disease: assessment of variability in pathologic interpretations. Mod Pathol 1998; 11(6):560–5.

48. Brunt EM, Neuschwander-Tetri BA, Oliver D, et al. Nonalcoholic steatohepatitis: histologic features and clinical correlations with 30 blinded biopsy specimens. Hum Pathol 2004;35:1070–82.

49. Kleiner DE, Brunt EM, Van Natta M, et al. Design and validation of a histologic scoring system for nonalcoholic fatty liver disease. Hepatology 2005;41: 1313–21.

50. Baldridge AD, Perez-Atayde AR, Graeme-Cooke F, et al. Idiopathic steatohepatitis in childhood: a multicenter retrospective study. J Pediatr 1995;127(5):700–4.

51. Schwimmer JB, Behling C, Newbury R, et al. Histopathology of pediatric nonalcoholic fatty liver disease. Hepatology 2005;42(3):641–9.

52. Wieckowska A, McCullough AJ, Feldstein AE. Noninvasive diagnosis and monitoring of nonalcoholic steatohepatitis: present and future. Hepatology 2007;46: 582–9.

53. Wieckowska A, Zein NN, Yerian LM, et al. In vivo assessment of liver cell apoptosis as a novel biomarker of disease severity in nonalcoholic fatty liver disease. Hepatology 2006;44:27–33.

54. Younossi ZM, Jarrar M, Nugent C, et al. A novel diagnostic biomarker panel for obesity-related nonalcoholic steatohepatitis (NASH). Obes Surg 2008 May 24.

55. Bedogni G, Bellentani S, Miglioli L, et al. The fatty liver index: a simple and accurate predictor of hepatic steatosis in the general population. BMC Gastroenterol 2006;6:33–9.

56. Ratziu V, Massard J, Charlotte F, et al. Diagnostic value of biochemical markers (FibroTest-FibroSURE) for the prediction of liver fibrosis in patients with nonalcoholic fatty liver disease. BMC Gastroenterol 2006;6:6.

57. Poynard T, Ratziu V, Naveau S, et al. The diagnostic value of biomarkers (SteatoTest) for the prediction of liver steatosis. Comp Hepatol 2005;4:10–24.

58. Ratziu V, Massard J, Charlotte F, et al. Diagnostic value of biochemical markers (FibroTest-FibroSURE) for the prediction of liver fibrosis in patients with nonalcoholic fatty liver disease. BMC Gastroenterol 2006;6:34.

59. Wai CT, Greenson JK, Fontana RJ, et al. A simple noninvasive index can predict both significant fibrosis and cirrhosis in patients with chronic hepatitis C. Hepatology 2003;38:518–26.

60. Cales P, Oberti F, Michalak S, et al. A novel panel of blood markers to assess the degree of liver fibrosis. Hepatology 2005;42:1373–81.

61. Angulo P, Hui JM, Marchesini G, et al. The NAFLD fibrosis score: a noninvasive system that accurately identifies liver fibrosis in patients with NAFLD. Hepatology 2007;45:846–54.

62. Rosenberg WM, Voelker M, Thiel R, et al. Serum markers detect the presence of liver fibrosis: a cohort study. Gastroenterology 2004;127:1704–13.

63. Guha IN, Parkes J, Roderick P, et al. Noninvasive markers of fibrosis in nonalcoholic fatty liver disease: validating the European liver fibrosis panel and exploring simple markers. Hepatology 2008;47:455–60.

64. Stewart KJ, Bacher AC, Turner K, et al. Exercise and risk factors associated with metabolic syndrome in older adults. Am J Prev Med 2005;28:9–18.

65. Palmer M, Schaffner F. Effect of weight reduction on hepatic abnormalities in overweight patients. Gastroenterology 1990;99:1408–13.

66. Andersen T, Gluud C, Franzmann ME, et al. Hepatic effects of dietary weight loss in morbidly obese subjects. J Hepatol 1991;12:224–9.

67. Ueno T, Suguwara J, Sujaku K, et al. Therapeutic effects of restricted diet and exercise in obese patients with fatty liver. J Hepatol 1997;27:103–7.

68. Harris RB, Kor H. Insulin insensitivity is rapidly reversed in rats by reducing dietary fat from 40 to 30% of energy. J Nutr 1992;122:1811–22.

69. Silberbauer CJ, Jacober B, Langhans W. Dietary fat level and short-term effects of a high-fat meal on food intake and metabolism. Ann Nutr Metab 1998;42: 75–89.

70. Oakes ND, Cooney GJ, Camilleri S, et al. Mechanisms of liver and muscle insulin resistance induced by chronic high-fat feeding. Diabetes 1997;46:1768–74.

71. Hallfrisch J, Facn, Behall KM. Mechanisms of the effects of grains on insulin and glucose responses. J Am Coll Nutr 2000;19:320S–5S.

72. Song YJ, Sawamura M, Ikeda K, et al. Soluble dietary fiber improves insulin sensitivity by increasing muscle GLUT-4 content in stroke prone spontaneously hypertensive rats. Clin Exp Pharmacol Physiol 2000;27:41–5.

73. Vajro P, Fontanella A, Perna C, et al. Persistent hyperaminotransferasemia resolving after weight reduction in obese children. J Pediatr 1994;125:239–41.

74. Harrison SA, Fincke C, Helinski D, et al. A pilot study of orlistat treatment in obese, non-alcoholic steatohepatitis patients. Aliment Pharmacol Ther 2004; 20:623–8.

75. Sabuncu T, Nazligul Y, Karaoglanoglu M, et al. The effects of sibutramine and orlistat on the ultrasonographic finding, insulin resistance and liver enzymes in obese patients with non-alcoholic steatohepatitis. Rom J Gastroenterol 2003; 12:189–92.

76. Gary-Bobo M, Elachouri G, Gallas JF, et al. Rimonabant reduces obesity-associated hepatic steatosis and features of metabolic syndrome in obese Zucker fa/fa rats. Hepatology 2007;46(1):122–9.

77. Rafiq N, Younossi ZM. Effects of weight loss on nonalcoholic fatty liver disease. Semin Liver Dis 2008;28(4):427–33.

78. Dixon JB, Bhathal PS, Hughes NR, et al. Nonalcoholic fatty liver disease: improvement in liver histological analysis with weight loss. Hepatology 2004; 39:1647–54.

79. Sjostrom L, Lindroos AK, Peltonen M, et al. Lifestyle, diabetes, and cardiovascular risk factors 10 years after bariatric surgery. N Engl J Med 2004;351: 2683–93.

80. Maggard MA, Shugarman LR, Suttorp M, et al. Meta-analysis: surgical treatment of obesity. Ann Intern Med 2005;142(7):547–59.

81. Bugianesi E, Gentilcore E, Nanini R, et al. A randomized controlled trial of metformin versus vitamin E or prescriptive diet in nonalcoholic fatty liver disease. Am J Gastroenterol 2005;100:1082–90.

82. Nair S, Diehl AM, Wiseman M, et al. Metformin in the treatment of non-alcoholic steatohepatitis: a pilot open label trial. Aliment Pharmacol Ther 2004;20:23–8.

83. Murase K, Odaka H, Suzuki M, et al. Pioglitazone time-dependently reduces tumour necrosis factor-alpha level in muscle and improves metabolic abnormalities in fatty rats. Diabetologia 1998;41:257–64.

84. Shimizu H, Tsuchiya T, Sato N, et al. Troglitazone reduces plasma leptin concentration but increases hunger in NIDDM patients. Diabetes Care 1998; 21:1470–4.

85. Neuschwander-Tetri BA, Brunt EM, Wehmeier KR, et al. Improved nonalcoholic steatohepatitis after 48 weeks of treatment with the PPAR-γ ligand rosiglitazone. Hepatology 2003;38(4):1008–17.

86. Ratziu V, Giral P, Jacqueminet S, et al. Rosiglitazone for nonalcoholic steatohepatitis: one-year results of the randomized placebo-controlled Fatty Liver Improvement with Rosiglitazone Therapy (FLIRT) Trial. Gastroenterology 2008;135(1):100–10.

87. Nathan DM. Rosiglitazone and cardiotoxicity—weighing the evidence. N Engl J Med 2007;357(1):64–6.

88. Grey A, Bolland M, Gamble G, et al. The peroxisome proliferator-activated receptor-agonist rosiglitazone decreases bone formation and bone mineral density in healthy postmenopausal women: a randomized, controlled trial. J Clin Endocrinol Metab 2007;92:1305–10.

89. Promrat K, Lutchman G, Uwaifo GI, et al. A pilot study of pioglitazone treatment for nonalcoholic steatohepatitis. Hepatology 2004;39:188–96.
90. Kiyici M, Gulten M, Gurel S, et al. Ursodeoxycholic acid and atorvastatin in the treatment of nonalcoholic steatohepatitis. Can J Gastroenterol 2003;17: 713–8.
91. Hatzitolios A, Savopoulos C, Lazaraki G, et al. Efficacy of omega-3 fatty acids, atorvastatin and orlistat in non-alcoholic fatty liver disease with dyslipidemia. Indian J Gastroenterol 2004;23:131–4.
92. Rallidis LS, Drakoulis CK, Parasi AS. Pravastatin in patients with nonalcoholic steatohepatitis: results of a pilot study. Atherosclerosis 2004;174:193–6.
93. Gomez-Dominguez E, Gisbert JP, Moreno-Monteagudo JA, et al. A pilot study of atorvastatin treatment in dyslipid, non-alcoholic fatty liver patients. Aliment Pharmacol Ther 2006;23:1643–7.
94. Ekstedt M, Franzen LE, Mathiesen UL, et al. Statins in non-alcoholic fatty liver disease and chronically elevated enzymes: a histopathological follow-up study. J Hepatol 2007;47:135–41.
95. Basaranoglu M, Acbay O, Sonsuz A. A controlled trial of gemfibrozil in the treatment of patients with nonalcoholic steatohepatitis [letter]. J Hepatol 1999; 31(2):384.
96. Laurin J, Lindor KD, Crippin JS, et al. Ursodeoxycholic acid or clofibrate in the treatment of non-alcohol-induced steatohepatitis: a pilot study. Hepatology 1996;23(6):1464–7.
97. Hasegawa T, Yoneda M, Nakamura K, et al. Plasma transforming growth factor—beta 1 level and efficacy of alpha-tocopherol in patients with non-alcoholic steatohepatitis: a pilot study. Aliment Pharmacol Ther 2001;15:1667–72.
98. Lavine JE. Vitamin E treatment of nonalcoholic steatohepatitis in children: a pilot study. J Pediatr 2001;136(6):734–8.
99. Vajro P, Mandalto C, Franzese A, et al. Vitamin treatment in pediatric obesity-related liver disease: a randomized study. J Pediatr Gastroenterol Nutr 2004; 38:48–55.
100. Kugelmas M, Hill DB, Vivian B, et al. Cytokines and NASH: a pilot study of the effects of lifestyle modification and vitamin E. Hepatology 2003;38: 413–9.
101. Harrison SA, Torgerson S, Hayashi P, et al. Vitamin E and vitamin C treatment improves fibrosis in patients with nonalcoholic steatohepatitis. Am J Gastroenterol 2003;98(11):2485–90.
102. Abdelmalek MF, Angulo P, Jorgensen RA, et al. Betaine, a promising new agent for patients with nonalcoholic steatohepatitis: results of a pilot study. Am J Gastroenterol 2001;96:2711–7.
103. Lindor KD, Kowdley KV, Heathcote EJ, et al. Ursodeoxycholic acid for treatment of nonalcoholic steatohepatitis: results of a randomized trial. Hepatology 2004; 39:770–8.
104. Yokohama S, Yoneda M, Haneda M, et al. Therapeutic efficacy of an angiotensin II receptor antagonist in patients with non alcoholic steatohepatitis. Hepatology 2004;40:1222–5.
105. Satapathy SK, Garg S, Chauhan R, et al. Beneficial effects of tumor necrosis factor-alpha inhibition by pentoxifylline on clinical, biochemical, and metabolic parameters of patients with nonalcoholic steatohepatitis. Am J Gastroenterol 2004;99:1946–52.
106. Adams LA, Zien CO, Angulo P, et al. A pilot trial of pentoxifylline in nonalcoholic steatohepatitis. Am J Gastroenterol 2004;99:2365–8.

107. Loguercio C, Federico A, Tuccillo C, et al. Beneficial effect of a probiotic VSL#3 on parameters of liver dysfunction in chronic liver diseases. J Clin Gastroenterol 2005;39(6):540–3.
108. Hazama Y, Matsuhisa M, Ohtoshi K, et al. Beneficial effects of nateglinide on insulin resistance in type 2 diabetes. Diabetes Res Clin Pract 2006;71(3):251–5.

Management of Alcoholic Liver Disease

Michael R. Lucey, MD, FRCPI

KEYWORDS

- Alcohol • Alcoholism • Cirrhosis • Hepatitis
- Abstinence

ADDICTION TO ALCOHOL

Addictions usually arise from pleasurable actions, and immediate gratification is the most common foundation for addiction. In the case of alcohol, the addictive state is divided into 2 classes within a spectrum: abuse, in which drinking is excessive but does not lead to many of the physical and social harmful consequences, and dependency, wherein drinking is continued despite physical and social injury. Ask an alcoholic person why they continue to drink, despite the obvious havoc alcohol is bringing to their lives and the lives of their family, and they will often say, "I drink because I like it."

The combination of gratification from the substance with the unwanted effects of the treatment, such as inconvenience of attending psychological therapy, embarrassment, financial disincentives, and ambivalence about the addictive behavior, can all contribute to addiction persisting. Consequently, substance abuse and addiction are disorders of remission and relapse.

Most reviews of alcoholic liver disease concentrate on treatment of the liver disease and do not address the underlying addiction. In practice, understanding the addiction is the key to understanding the continuum from alcoholic fatty liver to alcoholic cirrhosis. Furthermore, abstinence leads to resolution of alcoholic fatty liver and alcoholic hepatitis,[1,2] and, as shown by the classic studies of Powell and Klatskin, is associated with improved survival in alcoholic cirrhotic patients with decompensated liver function (**Fig. 1**).[3] Consequently, there is every reason to encourage alcoholic patients with liver disease to become abstinent.

When counseling an alcoholic patient, addiction specialists distinguish between a slip and a relapse.[4] A slip is a temporary return to drinking, which is recognized by the patient as potentially harmful, and leads to renewed efforts toward abstinence. A relapse suggests a more sustained resumption of drinking. These events are sometimes characterized as "harmful," "abusive," or "addictive drinking," whereas the term "recidivism" is abjured on account of its pejorative connotations.

Section of Gastroenterology and Hepatology, Department of Medicine, University of Wisconsin School of Medicine and Public Health, H6/516 CSC, 600 Highland Avenue, Madison, WI 53792, USA
E-mail address: mrl@medicine.wisc.edu

Clin Liver Dis 13 (2009) 267–275
doi:10.1016/j.cld.2009.02.003
1089-3261/09/$ – see front matter © 2009 Elsevier Inc. All rights reserved.

liver.theclinics.com

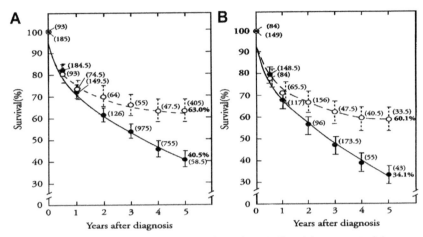

Fig. 1. Survival after diagnosis of alcoholic cirrhosis (n = 278) and from onset of decompensation (n = 233) according to continued alcohol use or abstinence. (*From* Powell WJ Jr., Klatskin G. Duration of survival in patients with Laennec's cirrhosis. Influence of alcohol withdrawal, and possible effects of recent changes in general management of the disease. Am J Med 1968;44(3):406–20; with permission.)

Treatment of addiction is directed at establishing and maintaining abstinence from the addictive behavior. Although continuing drinking that is less frequent or of reduced amounts is less than ideal, it is better than continuing harmful drinking. In contrast, in the world of hepatology, especially transplant, absolute abstinence is considered the only acceptable outcome, and any slip is judged to be a treatment failure. Many addiction specialists think that this is an unreasonable and unrealistic standard.[4] Furthermore, some specialists believe that this preoccupation with complete abstinence works against the best interests of the alcoholic patient with liver failure, since the patient may be frightened to seek help when he or she experiences a slip.[5] Recent long-term follow-up data suggest that relapse to harmful drinking affects survival after transplantation, whereas a history of a slip alone does not, further emphasizing the importance of this clinical distinction.[6]

TREATMENT OF ALCOHOLISM IN PATIENTS WITH LIVER DISEASE

Many alcoholic patients resume alcohol use despite life-threatening events such as variceal hemorrhage.[7] However, we understand only poorly what drives an alcoholic patient with liver disease to maintain abstinence, to slip and regain sobriety, or to relapse to harmful drinking. It is probable that alcoholic patients attending liver clinics or admitted as inpatients do not constitute a homogenous group but rather are a heterogeneous group determined in large part by selection biases. For example, both patients with alcoholic hepatitis and many alcoholic patients who present with acute variceal hemorrhage report recent alcohol use. In contrast, many alcoholic patients undergoing evaluation for liver transplantation usually report extended intervals of abstinence, often many years in duration.

The likelihood of alcoholic relapse and the motivation for treatment of alcoholism vary in these subgroups also. Thus, when a group of alcoholic patients undergoing transplant evaluation were compared with a matched group of alcoholics recruited to outpatient trials of alcoholism treatment, the liver clinic cohort reported significantly longer sobriety, little craving for alcohol, and low interest in treatment of alcoholism, whereas the group without liver disease reported significantly greater craving for alcohol and desire for treatment of alcoholism.[8] The perception that alcoholism is no longer a problem is common among alcoholic liver transplant recipients and limits their support for treatment.[9]

A comprehensive review of all interventions, psychological and medicinal, designed to ameliorate drinking behavior in alcoholic persons is beyond the scope of this review. Suffice it to say that few studies of treatment of alcohol abuse or dependence have included patients with alcoholic liver disease. Many use nuanced qualitative measures of reduced drinking, such as proportion of abstinent days and number of days with addictive drinking, as primary outcomes.[10,11] Harder endpoints, such as survival, or measures of liver health, such as the model for end-stage liver disease score, have rarely been assessed. There are few studies of psychological therapies directed at patients with significant liver injury. In one such example, the present author in conjunction with Robert Weinrieb of the University of Pennsylvania conducted a randomized study of motivational enhancement therapy (MET) versus treatment as usual in patients undergoing evaluation for liver transplantation (unpublished observations). Approximately 25% of subjects in either group admitted to some drinking in the period of follow-up, without any apparent benefit from MET.

As Garbutt and Flannery noted in 2007, "pharmacotherapy for alcoholism is undergoing a period of growth and scientific excitement."[12] However, there is a paucity of studies on the use of medications to deter patients with alcoholic liver injury or cirrhosis from drinking. Disulfiram, an antagonist of acetaldehyde dehydrogenase, has the longest period of approval for use in treating alcoholism. Hepatotoxicity and liver failure have been reported with use of disulfiram.[13,14] Furthermore, evidence of its efficacy is conflicting, and it has not been studied in a controlled fashion in patients with liver disease.

New drugs, such as oral or depot naltrexone and oral acamprosate, have been approved for use in alcoholic patients, whereas agents approved for other indications, such as baclofen or topiramate, have shown promise in controlling drinking behavior in alcoholic persons. Apart from baclofen, each of the studies mentioned below eschewed patients with known alcoholic cirrhosis. Concern remains about hepatotoxicity with naltrexone, which has a "black box" warning on this account. In the studies of agents designed to reduce the craving for alcohol described later, the observed effects have been modest reductions in total drinking, rather than substantial increases in total abstinence. Whether these qualitative effects would be accompanied by salutary effects on liver function, injury, or repair has not been shown, and therefore, it is too early to advocate their use in cirrhotic patients.

Several American multicenter clinical trials of the opioid receptor antagonist naltrexone have yielded conflicting results on drinking behavior.[15] For example, a study of 627 alcoholic subjects in the Veterans Affairs system failed to demonstrate an advantage in the treated group. In contrast, the Combined Pharmacotherapies and Behavioral Interventions (COMBINE) study, which comprised 1383 patients with alcohol dependence and at least 4 days of abstinence, showed a benefit for patients receiving naltrexone, but none for those receiving acamprosate (see below).[16,17] A multicenter study used a monthly injectable, extended-release naltrexone in comparison with placebo injections for 6 months in 624 alcohol subjects in whom alanine aminotransferase (ALT) or aspartate aminotransferase (AST) levels did not exceed 3 times the upper limit of normal ($>3 \cdot$ ULN) and found that depot naltrexone significantly decreased drinking.[18] A post hoc analysis of potential hepatotoxicity showed no significant differences in AST, ALT, or bilirubin levels between the study groups at study initiation or at subsequent assessments, whereas gamma-glutamyltransferase levels declined in the naltrexone group. Furthermore, there was no increase in frequency of high liver chemistry tests or hepatic-related adverse events in naltrexone-treated subjects who were drinking heavily throughout the study, in obese subjects, or in those taking nonsteroidal anti-inflammatory medicines.[19] In summary, although the data suggest that naltrexone may enhance sobriety, and the depot preparation, which promotes adherence at lower doses, appears safe in actively drinking alcoholics, neither preparation of naltrexone can be recommended for cirrhotic patients until they have been tested in this population.

In a large multicenter study, comparing acamprosate with placebo, acamprosate was associated with a modest improvement in days without drinking and in percentage of complete abstainers over a 1-year observation period.[20] Apart from mild diarrhea, there was no increase in side effects in the acamprosate subjects. It is interesting that the COMBINE study, mentioned above, failed to find a benefit of acamprosate in reducing drinking behavior in a study in which naltrexone was associated with a modest reduction in frequency and severity of drinking.[17]

Topiramate, which is approved as an anticonvulsant, has been studied in alcoholism. Although its exact mechanism of action is unknown, it is proposed to reduce alcohol's reinforcing influence on continued drinking through enhancement of γ-aminobutyric acid and inhibition of glutaminergic central neurologic pathways. Topiramate has been shown to improve drinking outcomes in a randomized, multicenter, placebo-controlled study lasting 14 weeks among 371 alcohol-dependent subjects who had normal liver chemistries and were not known to have cirrhosis.[21] Further analysis of this study showed a minor improvement in serum aminotransferase levels in the topiramate-treated cohort.[22]

Addolorato and co-workers[23] reported a randomized clinical trial in which 84 patients with alcoholic cirrhosis received oral baclofen or placebo for 12 weeks with 4 weeks' follow-up. They showed that 30 of 42 (71%) of the baclofen-treated patients achieved and maintained abstinence compared with only 12 of 42 (29%) in the placebo arm. The study is exceptional in that it enrolled patients with alcoholic cirrhosis, who are usually excluded from such studies. It will be necessary to see further studies such as this in patients with known liver disease, with greater power, and longer duration of treatment to define baclofen's role.

TREATMENT OF ALCOHOLIC HEPATITIS

Corticosteroids have become the standard of care in selected patients with alcoholic hepatitis. Selected patients should have severe alcoholic hepatitis, as shown by a Maddrey discriminant function greater than or equal to 32, no or controlled infection, and no major contraindication to use of corticosteroids. This consensus is based on a number of key publications. Principal among them is the reanalysis by Mathurin and colleagues[24] of the original data from 3 prior randomized, clinical trials of prednisolone in patients with acute alcoholic hepatitis. All subjects had a Maddrey discriminant function greater than or equal to 32. At 28 days, 113 corticosteroid patients had significantly higher survival (84.6% ± 3.4%) compared with a survival of 65.1% ± 4.8% in 102 placebo-treated patients. In multivariate analysis, age ($P = .0001$), serum creatinine ($P<.002$), and corticosteroid treatment ($P = .002$) were independent prognostic variables.

In a series of important papers, Mathurin's group has defined a stopping rule to determine whether to continue or stop corticosteroids. In 2003, they observed that patients who had a reduction in total bilirubin within the first 7 days of treatment had a good

6-month survival, whereas those who did not had a very poor outcome.[25] They have further refined this observation to form the so-called Lille model, which combines 6 reproducible variables (age, renal insufficiency, albumin, prothrombin time, bilirubin, and evolution of bilirubin at day 7) to provide a very accurate prognostic marker of 6-month survival.[26] The formula is available online at http://www.lillemodel.com. Unfortunately, the anticipated survival is only 25% among patients with alcoholic hepatitis treated for 7 days compared with a 6-month survival of 85% $\pm$ 2.5% in the remainder. The recommendation is to start corticosteroids in patients with severe alcoholic hepatitis who are not septic, and then assess at day 7. If the Lille score is less than 0.45, the patient should complete 28 days of corticosteroid therapy. If the Lille score is above the threshold, the corticosteroids should be stopped at day 7. It has not been determined whether it is better to taper or stop the corticosteroids without a taper. Although the Lille score is a useful parameter, it underscores the dire outcome in those patients who fail to respond to the first 7 days of corticosteroid therapy.

A Cochrane systematic review concluded that the available evidence does not support the use of anabolic-androgenic steroids in patients with severe alcoholic hepatitis.[27]

Two anti-tumor necrosis factor alpha (TNF-α) agents have been studied in patients with alcoholic hepatitis: infliximab and etanercept. Infliximab is a chimeric, monoclonal antibody to TNF-α. A recent randomized, controlled trial comparing intravenous infusion of infliximab plus prednisone with placebo plus prednisolone in patients with severe alcoholic hepatitis was stopped prematurely by the independent data safety monitoring board on account of a significantly greater number of severe infections and a nonsignificant increase in deaths in the infliximab plus prednisolone cohort.[28] Etanercept, which consists of 2 units of human recombinant, soluble TNF-α receptor type 11 (p 75) fused with the Fc domain of human IgG1, binds soluble TNF-α. Although etanercept appeared to increase short-term survival in a small pilot study,[29] a more recent formal, randomized, clinical trial in patients with severe alcoholic hepatitis, conducted by the same investigators, failed to confirm this benefit.

Pentoxifylline is a phosphodiesterase inhibitor approved for the treatment of intermittent claudication. The modulation of the transcription of the TNF-α gene is one putative mechanism for the salutary effect of pentoxifylline in alcoholic hepatitis, although other actions on vascular function are also of potential importance. Akriviadis and colleagues[30] compared the effect of either pentoxifylline (400 mg orally 3 times daily for 4 weeks) or placebo in 101 patients with severe alcoholic hepatitis. Patients with active gastrointestinal hemorrhage, systemic infection, or severe cardiopulmonary disease, as well as patients who appeared to be improving rapidly or patients with features of advanced cirrhosis were excluded. Corticosteroids were not used. The primary end points were 28-day mortality or progression to hepatorenal syndrome. Twelve (24.5%) of the 49 pentoxifylline patients and 24 (46.1%) of the 52 placebo patients died during the initial hospitalization. Hepatorenal syndrome was implicated as a cause of death in 6 of 12 deaths (50%) in the treated group and 22 of 24 deaths (91.7%) among the placebo patients. Thus, Akriviadis' study provides the best evidence to date that pentoxifylline improves mortality in patients with alcoholic hepatitis. In contrast, Mathurin and colleagues[31] found that adding pentoxifylline as a rescue agent was ineffective in patients with severe alcoholic hepatitis who did not respond to initial corticosteroid therapy.

Although nutritional support improves nutritional status, it does not decrease early mortality in patients with alcoholic hepatitis.[32]

Despite the evidence that alcoholic liver disease is associated with enhanced oxidative stress, studies have failed to show that antioxidants confer any benefit in alcoholic hepatitis or alcoholic cirrhosis.[33,34]

TREATMENT OF CIRRHOSIS

Therapeutic approaches to the common complications of alcoholic cirrhosis, such as ascites, variceal hemorrhage, and encephalopathy, are addressed elsewhere in this issue. As already discussed, the most common cause of decompensation of alcoholic cirrhosis is recent excessive use of alcohol. Similarly, the most important therapeutic factor in recovery is abstinence, and the most common reason for failure of recovery is that the patient resumes drinking.[35] The progression of fibrosis in alcoholic patients is exacerbated by the presence of viral hepatitis B or C.[36,37] Although the treatment of viral hepatitis has not been studied extensively in patients with alcoholism and liver disease, it is possible that antiviral therapy would arrest the progression of fibrosis in some patients.

Several medications, including propylthiouracil (PTU), colchicine, S-adenosylmethionine (SAMe), milk thistle or silymarin, and polyenylphosphatidylcholine, have been proposed for treatment of alcoholic fibrosis and cirrhosis. Although favorable clinical trial results have been reported for PTU, colchicine, and SAMe, none has become established as a standard therapy.[38–40] The reasons differ depending on the agent under review. Regarding PTU, despite the thoughtful advocacy of the authors, including showing that hypothyroidism is rare and that PTU improves mortality even when the patient continues to drink occasionally, fear of side effects has limited the acceptance of this agent.[41] Colchicine has been the focus of a well-designed placebo-controlled multicenter study in 549 patients with advanced alcoholic cirrhosis that failed to reproduce the previously reported favorable effect on mortality.[42] In a study limited by relative lack of power, administration of SAME or placebo to 123 patients with alcoholic cirrhosis for 2 years showed a trend for improved survival, which was not statistically significant.[40] Well-designed clinical trials using silymarin or phosphatidylcholine have been reported in the treatment of alcoholic liver disease.[43,44] Silymarin administered to alcoholic patients with liver cirrhosis showed no effect on either survival or the clinical course. Polyenylphosphatidylcholine administered to alcoholic patients with liver fibrosis did not improve survival nor prevent the progression of fibrosis.

LIVER TRANSPLANTATION

Liver transplantation has become an accepted therapy for selected patients with liver failure or hepatocellular carcinoma associated with alcoholic cirrhosis.[45] In addition to the standard elements of liver transplantation, these patients undergo careful assessment of psychosocial health and their capacity to maintain abstinence from future alcohol use. Many programs use an arbitrary minimal criterion of 6 months' abstinence as a requirement for placement on the transplant waiting list, although the utility of this "rule" as a predictor of future drinking has been challenged. Post-transplant graft and patient survival for alcoholic patients is similar to that for nonalcoholic liver transplant recipient, although patients who return to abusive drinking are at risk of liver injury and reduced survival in the longer term.[6]

REFERENCES

1. Teli MR, Day CP, Burt AD, et al. Determinants of progression to cirrhosis or fibrosis in pure alcoholic fatty liver. Lancet 1995;346(8981):987–90.
2. Lischner MW, Alexander JF, Galambos JT. Natural history of alcoholic hepatitis. I. The acute disease. Am J Dig Dis 1971;16(6):481–94.

3. Powell WJ Jr, Klatskin G. Duration of survival in patients with Laennec's cirrhosis. Influence of alcohol withdrawal, and possible effects of recent changes in general management of the disease. Am J Med 1968;44(3):406–20.
4. Fuller RK. Definition and diagnosis of relapse to drinking. Liver Transpl Surg 1997; 3(3):258–62.
5. Weinrieb RM, Van Horn DH, McLellan AT, et al. Interpreting the significance of drinking by alcohol-dependent liver transplant patients: fostering candor is the key to recovery. Liver Transpl 2000;6(6):769–76.
6. Pfitzmann R, Schwenzer J, Rayes N, et al. Long-term survival and predictors of relapse after orthotopic liver transplantation for alcoholic liver disease. Liver Transpl 2007;13:197–205.
7. Lucey MR, Connor JT, Boyer TD, et al. DIVERT Study Group. Alcohol consumption by cirrhotic subjects: patterns of use and effects on liver function. Am J Gastro-enterol 2008;103(7):1698–706.
8. Weinrieb RM, Van Horn DH, McLellan AT, et al. Drinking behavior and motivation for treatment among alcohol-dependent liver transplant candidates. J Addict Dis 2001;20(2):105–19.
9. Weinrieb RM, Van Horn DH, McLellan AT, et al. Alcoholism treatment after liver transplantation: lessons learned from a clinical trial that failed. Psychosomatics 2001;42(2):110–6.
10. Matching alcoholism treatments to client heterogeneity: project MATCH three-year drinking outcomes. Alcohol Clin Exp Res 1998;22(6):1300–11.
11. Garbutt JC, West SL, Carey TS, et al. Pharmacological treatment of alcohol dependence: a review of the evidence. JAMA 1999;281:1318–25.
12. Garbutt JC, Flannery B. Baclofen for alcoholism. Lancet 2007;370(9603):1884–5.
13. Vanjak D, Samuel D, Gosset F, et al. Fulminant hepatitis induced by disulfiram in a patient with alcoholic cirrhosis. Survival after liver transplantation. Gastroenterol Clin Biol 1989;13:1075–8.
14. Forns X, Caballería J, Bruguera M, et al. Disulfiram-induced hepatitis. Report of four cases and review of the literature. J Hepatol 1994;21:853–7.
15. Anton RF. Naltrexone for the management of alcohol dependence. N Engl J Med 2008;359:715–21.
16. Krystal JH, Cramer JA, Krol WF, et al. Naltrexone in the treatment of alcohol dependence. N Engl J Med 2001;345:1734–9.
17. Anton RF, O'Malley SS, Ciraulo DA, et al. Combined pharmacotherapies and behavioral interventions for alcohol dependence: the COMBINE study: a random-ized controlled trial. JAMA 2006;295:2003–17.
18. Garbutt JC, Kranzler HR, O'Malley SS, et al. Vivitrex Study Group. Efficacy and tolerability of long-acting injectable naltrexone for alcohol dependence: a randomized controlled trial. JAMA 2005;293:1617–25.
19. Lucey MR, Silverman BL, Illeperuma A, et al. Hepatic safety of once-monthly injectable extended-release naltrexone administered to actively drinking alco-holics. Alcohol Clin Exp Res 2008;32:498–504.
20. Whitworth AB, Fischer F, Lesch OM, et al. Comparison of acamprosate and placebo in long-term treatment of alcohol dependence. Lancet 1996; 347(9013):1438–42.
21. Johnson BA, Rosenthal N, Capece JA, et al. Topiramate for Alcoholism Advisory Board; Topiramate for Alcoholism Study Group. Topiramate for treating alcohol dependence: a randomized controlled trial. JAMA 2007;298(14):1641–51.
22. Johnson BA, Rosenthal N, Capece JA, et al. Topiramate for Alcoholism Advisory Board; Topiramate for Alcoholism Study Group. Improvement of physical health

and quality of life of alcohol-dependent individuals with topiramate treatment: US multisite randomized controlled trial. Arch Intern Med 2008;168(11):1188–99.

23. Addolorato G, Leggio L, Ferrulli A, et al. Effectiveness and safety of baclofen for maintenance of alcohol abstinence in alcohol-dependent patients with liver cirrhosis: randomised, double-blind controlled study. Lancet 2007;370(9603): 1915–22.

24. Mathurin P, Mendenhall CL, Carithers RL Jr, et al. Corticosteroids improve short-term survival in patients with severe alcoholic hepatitis (AH): individual data analysis of the last three randomized placebo controlled double blind trials of corticosteroids in severe AH. J Hepatol 2002;36:480–7.

25. Mathurin P, Abdelnour M, Ramond MJ, et al. Early change in bilirubin levels is an important prognostic factor in severe alcoholic hepatitis treated with predniso-lone. Hepatology 2003;38:1363–9.

26. Louvet A, Naveau S, Abdelnour M, et al. The Lille model: a new tool for thera-peutic strategy in patients with severe alcoholic hepatitis treated with steroids. Hepatology 2007;45:1348–54.

27. Rambaldi A, Iaquinto G, Gluud C. Anabolic-androgenic steroids for alcoholic liver disease. Cochrane Database Syst Rev 2003;(1):CD003045.

28. Naveau S, Chollet-Martin S, Dharancy S, et al. Foie-Alcool group of the Associa-tion Francaise pour l'Etude du Foie. A double-blind randomized controlled trial of infliximab associated with prednisolone in acute alcoholic hepatitis. Hepatology 2004;39:1390–7.

29. Menon KV, Stadheim L, Kamath PS, et al. A pilot study of the safety and tolera-bility of etanercept in patients with alcoholic hepatitis. Am J Gastroenterol 2004;99:255–60.

30. Akriviadis E, Botla R, Briggs W, et al. Pentoxifylline improves short-term survival in severe acute alcoholic hepatitis: a double-blind, placebo-controlled trial. Gastro-enterology 2000;119:1637–48.

31. Louvet A, Diaz E, Dharancy S, et al. Early switch to pentoxifylline in patients with severe alcoholic hepatitis is inefficient in non-responders to corticosteroids. J Hepatol 2008;48:465–70.

32. Stickel F, Hoehn B, Schuppan D, et al. Nutritional therapy in alcoholic liver disease. Aliment Pharmacol Ther 2003;18:357–73.

33. Mezey E, Potter JJ, Rennie-Tankersley L, et al. A randomized placebo controlled trial of vitamin E for alcoholic hepatitis. J Hepatol 2004;1:40–6.

34. Stewart S, Prince M, Bassendine M, et al. A randomized trial of antioxidant therapy alone or with corticosteroids in acute alcoholic hepatitis. J Hepatol 2007;47:277–83.

35. Veldt BJ, Lainé F, Guillygomarc'h A, et al. Indication of liver transplantation in severe alcoholic liver cirrhosis: quantitative evaluation and optimal timing. J Hep-atol 2002;36:93–8.

36. Frieden TR, Ozick L, McCord C, et al. Chronic liver disease in central Harlem: the role of alcohol and viral hepatitis. Hepatology 1999;29:883–8.

37. Corrao G, Aricò S. Independent and combined action of hepatitis C virus infec-tion and alcohol consumption on the risk of symptomatic liver cirrhosis. Hepatol-ogy 1998;27:914–9.

38. Orrego H, Blake JE, Blendis LM, et al. Long-term treatment of alcoholic liver disease with propylthiouracil. N Engl J Med 1987;317:1421–7.

39. Kershenobich D, Vargas F, Garcia-Tsao G, et al. Colchicine in the treatment of cirrhosis of the liver. N Engl J Med 1988;318:1709–13.

40. Mato JM, Cámara J, Fernández de Paz J, et al. S-adenosylmethionine in alcoholic liver cirrhosis: a randomized, placebo-controlled, double-blind, multicenter clinical trial. J Hepatol 1999;30:1081–9.
41. Orrego H, Blake JE, Blendis LM, et al. Long-term treatment of alcoholic liver disease with propylthiouracil. Part 2: influence of drop-out rates and of continued alcohol consumption in a clinical trial. J Hepatol 1994;20:343–9.
42. Morgan TR, Weiss DG, Nemchausky B, et al. Colchicine treatment of alcoholic cirrhosis: a randomized, placebo-controlled clinical trial of patient survival. Gastroenterology 2005;128:882–90.
43. Pares A, Planas R, Torres M, et al. Effects of silymarin in alcoholic patients with cirrhosis of the liver: results of a controlled, double-blind, randomized and multicenter trial. J Hepatol 1998;4:615–21.
44. Lieber CS, Weiss DG, Groszmann R, et al. For the Veterans Affairs Cooperative Study 391 Group. II. Veterans Affairs Cooperative Study of polyenylphosphatidylcholine in alcoholic liver disease. Alcohol Clin Exp Res 2003;27:1765–72.
45. Lucey MR. Liver transplantation for alcoholic liver disease. Clin Liver Dis 2007;11:283–9.

Drug-Induced Hepatotoxicity or Drug-Induced Liver Injury

Aaron J. Pugh, DO[a], Ashutosh J. Barve, MD, PhD[b], Keith Falkner, PhD[b],
Mihir Patel, MD[a], Craig J. McClain, MD[a,c,d,]*

KEYWORDS

- Drugs • Liver injury • Antibiotics • Alternative medicine
- Antiretroviral

Drug-induced hepatotoxicity or drug-induced liver injury (DILI) is an important cause of liver disease with an incidence of between 1 in 1,000 and 1 in 100,000 in patients taking therapeutic doses of medications.[1] Drug-induced hepatotoxicity is believed to be underreported, and the incidence of drug-induced hepatotoxicity is largely underestimated in the general population.[2] Liver toxicity is the most common form of adverse drug reaction resulting in aborted drug development or withdrawal after licensing. Drugs that are hepatotoxic may exhibit characteristic clinical signatures. These characteristics include patterns of liver test abnormalities, latency of symptom onset, presence or absence of immune hypersensitivity, and the course of the reaction after drug withdrawal.[3]

Drug-induced hepatotoxicity accounts for more than 50% of cases of acute liver failure, with acetaminophen the most frequent cause in the United States. Fatal outcomes are frequent in patients with acute liver injury due to drugs other than acetaminophen overdose.[4] DILI accounts for almost 10% of liver transplants in some centers. Development of jaundice in combination with elevated aminotransferases in patients with DILI is associated with an estimated mortality rate of 10%.[5] Early

---

Funding support: Research support was provided by the National Institutes of Health (McClain) and the VA (McClain).

[a] Department of Medicine, University of Louisville School of Medicine, 550 South Jackson Street, Louisville, KY 40292, USA
[b] Division of Gastroenterology/Hepatology, Department of Medicine, University of Louisville School of Medicine, 550 South Jackson Street, Louisville, KY 40292, USA
[c] Department of Pharmacology and Toxicology, University of Louisville School of Medicine, 550 South Jackson Street, Louisville, KY 40292, USA
[d] Louisville VAMC, Louisville, KY 40206, USA
* Corresponding author. Department of Medicine, University of Louisville School of Medicine, 550 South Jackson Street, Louisville, KY 40292.
E-mail address: cjmccl01@gwise.louisville.edu (C.J. McClain).

Clin Liver Dis 13 (2009) 277–294
doi:10.1016/j.cld.2009.02.008
1089-3261/09/$ – see front matter. Published by Elsevier Inc.

liver.theclinics.com

detection of acute liver failure with prompt referral to a liver transplant center for transplant workup is essential.

Review articles addressing drug-induced hepatotoxicity generally cover either mechanisms of injury or common drugs causing toxicity. In this article, important concepts and new advances in drug-induced hepatotoxicity are reviewed, taking the latter approach of reviewing specific drugs. A brief overview of drug metabolism and mechanisms of hepatotoxicity is provided, and classes of drugs causing hepatotoxicity are reviewed, including lipid lowering agents, oral hypoglycemics, psychotropics, antiretrovirals, antibiotics, acetaminophen, and complementary and alternative medicine agents.

OVERVIEW OF DRUG METABOLISM AND TOXICITY

Most oral drugs absorbed from the gastrointestinal tract are lipophilic and water insoluble. These drugs must undergo hepatic metabolism by way of a phase I reaction to allow them to become hydrophilic. This phase I reaction is accomplished by oxidation, reduction, or hydrolysis. These reactions are catalyzed primarily by the cytochrome P450 superfamily of enzymes.[6]

The hydrophilic metabolites from phase I metabolism then undergo phase II reactions in which a polar group is added to the metabolite to allow for excretion. These reactions are mainly performed by conjugation with glutathione, glucuronic acid, or sulfate to produce a more water-soluble product recognized by drug transporters and excreted in either urine or bile.[7]

Drug metabolism can be affected by multiple factors, such as diet, age, genetics, underlying liver disease, and the presence of other drugs.[8] These factors must be considered when prescribing a possibly hepatotoxic drug to a patient who is at increased risk for developing drug-induced hepatotoxicity.[9] **Table 1** provides selected examples of drugs, the toxicity of which may be influenced by external/environmental factors.

Table 1 External/environmental factors and risk for DILI		
Factor	**Factor Modifier**	**Examples**
Age	Children, ↑ hepatotoxicity	Valproic acid, salicylates
	>60 y, ↑ hepatotoxicity	Isoniazid, halothane
Gender	Men, ↑ hepatotoxicity	Azathioprine
	Women, ↑ hepatotoxicity	Nitrofurantoin, halothane
Nutrition	Obesity, ↑ hepatotoxicity	Methotrexate
	Fasting, ↑ hepatotoxicity	Acetaminophen
Excessive ethyl alcohol	↑ hepatotoxicity	Acetaminophen, isoniazid
Dose	↑ blood levels → ↑ hepatotoxicity	Acetaminophen, aspirin
	Exposure dose, duration ↑ Hepatotoxicity	Methotrexate, vitamin A
Other drugs	↑ Hepatotoxicity	Rifampicin, pyrazinamide, and isoniazid
	↑ Hepatotoxicity	Other antiepileptics and valproic acid
Hepatitis C, B	↑ Hepatotoxicity	HAART therapy

Abbreviations: ↑, increased; →, leads to.

Drug-induced hepatotoxicity can manifest as either direct or idiosyncratic reactions. Direct hepatotoxicity is generally dose dependent. Idiosyncratic reactions are manifested after a delay or latency period ranging from 5 to 90 days after drug ingestion.[1] Direct or dose-dependent hepatotoxicity is reproducible and often has a predictable course. The period of time between initiation of a drug and hepatotoxicity is usually consistent from person to person for each drug. The dosage required to produce liver injury is also consistent from person to person. Drug-induced hepatotoxicity can present as a hepatocellular, cholestatic, or mixed picture. Dose-dependent toxicity can occur as a result of drug biotransformation by hepatocytes, catalyzed by cytochrome P450 enzymes, which generate additional toxic/reactive intermediates, acetaminophen being a classic example.[10] During hepatocellular injury, serum aminotransferases can be elevated several hundredfold with minimal elevation of alkaline phosphatase.[11] Many drugs that cause dose-dependent toxicity have a signature or expected pattern of injury.[9]

Most drug-induced hepatotoxicity is idiosyncratic and unpredictable rather than directly hepatotoxic. Idiosyncratic reactions can also be classified as hepatocellular, cholestatic, or mixed. These classifications are general terms and do not apply to all circumstances.[12] Idiosyncratic reactions can be divided into 2 main categories: metabolic or immunologic. Metabolic reactions may result from a specific genetic polymorphism resulting in the formation of a toxic metabolite.[13] These are considered idiosyncratic toxicities because the reaction caused by a specific genetic polymorphism is not reproducible from person to person. Immunologic reactions are hypersensitivity reactions to a specific drug. The immunologic response is often due to a drug–protein adduct in the liver. The reaction includes a delayed response and laboratory evidence of immunologic alterations. These hypersensitivities have features including mild fever, eosinophilia, atypical lymphocytosis, and liver infiltrates.[10] Other features can include granulocytopenia, thrombocytopenia, hemolytic anemia, Stevens-Johnson syndrome, and toxic epidermal necrolysis. The most definitive confirmation of a hypersensitivity reaction is a rapid positive rechallenge. This approach is not recommended and is rarely, if ever, justified.[3]

HEPATOTOXICITY CAUSED BY LIPID LOWERING AGENTS

Statins, or HMG-CoA reductase inhibitors, are widely prescribed for hyperlipidemia. Although statins cause a dose-related increase in transaminases, there is no clear evidence that they cause severe hepatotoxicity.[14] Statins as a class typically cause hepatocellular liver injury or mixed hepatocellular and cholestatic liver injury. Acute hepatic failure caused by statins is extremely rare, with an estimated incidence of 2 in 1 million patients treated with statins. With this small number, it is impossible to directly attribute liver failure to statin usage.[15,16] Moreover, statin hepatotoxicity is frequently asymptomatic and usually resolves after dose reduction or drug withdrawal.[17]

Pravastatin (not metabolized by cytochrome P450 enzymes) has been postulated to be less hepatotoxic than other statins metabolized by cytochrome P450 enzymes, although this concept has never been rigorously tested.[15,18] Pravastatin has been reported to cause an increase in transaminases, and has been reported as a cause of hepatic failure.[19]

There is no evidence that monitoring liver enzymes reduces the rate of hepatotoxicity with statins,[20] but patients should have their liver enzymes checked before initiation of statin therapy as many of these patients will have non–alcohol-related fatty liver disease.[16]

Ezetimibe lowers cholesterol by inhibiting intestinal absorption of cholesterol at the brush border of the small intestine. Ezetimibe has been shown to have a rate of adverse events similar to placebo when used as a sole agent. Ezetimibe and concomitant statin use has been shown to cause a slight elevation of transaminases compared with statin use alone.[21] The combination of simvistatin plus ezetimibe has recently been reported to induce acute liver failure in a 70-year-old Hispanic woman who subsequently required liver transplantation.[22]

Niacin, or nicotinic acid, is commonly used to increase high-density lipoprotein while reducing total cholesterol, low-density lipoprotein cholesterol, and triglycerides.[23,24] Niacin is available in 3 different preparations including immediate release (crystalline or IR), extended release (ER), and long acting (LA) preparations. All 3 preparations are available over-the-counter and by prescription. Niacin is known to cause hepatotoxicity in all preparations, with the LA preparation and the ER preparation implicated more frequently than the IR form.[25,26] Cholestatic injury has been reported,[27] but most hepatotoxicity is hepatocellular with multiple reported cases of acute liver failure.[28–30] However, elevated transaminases usually return to normal after withdrawal of nicotinic acid.[24]

The specific preparation of niacin determines the pathway for drug metabolism. Niacin is metabolized by conjugation forming nicotinuric acid, and by the nicotinamide pathway with the formation of hepatotoxic metabolites. The nicotinamide pathway is a high-affinity, low-capacity pathway that is quickly saturated by the IR niacin, preventing formation of the hepatotoxic metabolites. ER and LA niacin are slowly absorbed and metabolized by the nicotinamide pathway resulting in hepatotoxic metabolites.[31,32]

Fibrates are commonly prescribed medications for treatment of hypertriglyceridemia. A case has been reported of fenofibrate and raloxifene causing prolonged cholestasis.[33] Another case report in the Spanish literature describes gemfibrozil causing cholestatic hepatitis.[34]

ORAL HYPOGLYCEMICS

Thiazolidinediones (TZDs) are peroxisome proliferator-activated receptor γ agonists used as insulin-sensitizing drugs to treat diabetes mellitus. This class of drugs is a well-recognized cause of drug-induced hepatotoxicity. The first TZD, troglitazone, was withdrawn from the market in 2000 following 94 cases of liver failure.[35,36] There are 2 second generation TZDs on the market at the current time: rosiglitazone and pioglitazone. Both of these second generation TZDs are known to cause hepatotoxicity,[37–41] with rare reports of hepatic failure.[38–41] It is recommended that liver enzymes be determined before initiation of rosiglitazone or pioglitazone, and periodically after starting therapy.[42,43]

PSYCHOTROPICS

Selective serotonin reuptake inhibitors, serotonin-norepinephrine reuptake inhibitors, tricyclic antidepressants, and monoamine oxidase inhibitors are commonly prescribed medications for depression that have the potential to cause hepatotoxicity. Of the selective serotonin reuptake inhibitors, paroxetine has generated the greatest number of reports of hepatotoxicity.[44,45] Nefazodone, a serotonin-norepinephrine reuptake inhibitor, seems to have the greatest risk of severe hepatotoxicity and has a black box warning.[44,46]

Tolcapone, a catechol-O-methyl transferase inhibitor, is used to treat Parkinson's disease along with levodopa–carbidopa. In preclinical testing, no hepatotoxicity was detected, with only a 1% elevation of transaminases with the 100-mg dose versus placebo and 3% elevation of transaminases with the 200-mg dose versus placebo.[47] A retrospective analysis conducted in 2007 concluded that significant hepatotoxicity due to tolcapone is rare and often transient.[48] However, tolcapone carries a black box warning for acute liver failure, with reports of 3 cases of a fatal outcome.[49]

ANTIRETROVIRALS

Antiretroviral medications are widely used to treat HIV-infected patients. Three classes of antiretrovirals currently exist: nucleoside analogue reverse transcriptase inhibitors, nonnucleoside reverse transcriptase inhibitors, and protease inhibitors (PIs).[50] All 3 classes have been shown to cause severe hepatotoxicity in patients receiving highly active antiretroviral therapy (HAART).[51] Hepatotoxicity due to HAART is common, with up to 30% of patients on HAART experiencing World Health Organization grade 3 liver enzyme elevations.[52] Furthermore, hepatotoxicity from antiretroviral drugs leads to adverse patient outcomes either from acute hepatic failure, or, more commonly, AIDS following discontinuation of HAART.[53] Some of the more likely mechanisms of hepatotoxicity include proinflammatory cytokine production, mitochondrial toxicity, hypersensitivity reactions, steatosis and insulin resistance, increased immune response in hepatitis C or hepatitis B coinfected patients, and proteosome inhibition.[54–56] Hepatotoxicity caused by HAART is usually acute, often asymptomatic, and self-limited,[57] although acute hepatic failure has been reported with all 3 classes.[58–62] Some risk factors for hepatotoxicity include viral hepatitis coinfection with hepatitis C or hepatitis B, advanced liver disease, and elevated transaminases before the start of HAART.[51]

Didanosine (Videx EC) and stavudine (Zerit) are among the most commonly cited nucleoside analogue reverse transcriptase inhibitors causing hepatotoxicity.[51] Didanosine and stavudine are synthetic nucleoside analogues that have been reported to cause a rare, but potentially fatal, hepatic steatosis and lactic acidosis.[59,60] This is believed to be a result of inhibition of mitochondrial DNA polymerase γ, which is involved in the replication and repair of mitochondrial DNA with subsequent mitochondrial toxicity.[63] Didanosine and stavudine are known to cause elevations in transaminases and carry black box warnings due to fatal cases of lactic acidosis and severe hepatomegaly with steatosis.[59,60]

Nevirapine (Viramune) is a common nonnucleoside reverse transcriptase inhibitor causing hepatotoxicity.[51,61] Nevirapine binds directly to reverse transcriptase inhibiting polymerase activity. Nevirapine causes elevations in transaminases and carries a black box warning for fatal and nonfatal hepatotoxicity. Monitoring of liver enzymes for the first 18 weeks of therapy is recommended. Hepatic failure/hepatitis can be associated with signs of hypersensitivity including rash, fever, and eosinophilia.[61]

Ritonavir (Norvir) and tipranavir (Aptivus) are PIs known to cause hepatotoxicity and acute liver failure.[64,65] Hepatocellular liver injury and cholestasis have been reported with ritonavir.[64] The incidence of liver enzyme elevation with ritonavir is between 5% and 30% with an average onset between 2 and 6 months following drug initiation. Like ritonavir, tipranavir causes elevation of liver enzymes in 5% to 17% of patients.[65] It also carries a black box warning for hepatotoxicity with even fatal hepatic decompensation when used in combination with ritonavir.[65] In 2002, a study evaluating patients who were coinfected with HIV and hepatitis C and antiretroviral therapy with single versus dual protease inhibitors found no decrease in hepatotoxicity with the single protease inhibitor group compared with the dual protease inhibitor group.[66]

One mechanism of PI-dependent hepatotoxicity is believed to involve inhibition of proteosomal activity.[67] This leads to an increase in proteins such as the sterol regulatory element binding protein transcription factors, which are believed to play a role in the development of steatosis and lipodystrophy.[68] Another important consideration is that PIs are pregnane and xenobiotic receptor (PXR) ligands that induce CYP3A expression, are metabolized by CYP3A, and following metabolism can become mechanism-based inhibitors of CYP3A.[69] Thus, patients receiving PIs may display a highly variable drug metabolism profile with large differences in the ability to metabolize these and other drugs, and consequently idiosyncratic drug toxicity may be anticipated.[70] This toxicity can be further complicated in individuals receiving other drugs that are either metabolized by CYP3A or induce CYP3A expression. Particularly problematic are people who are HIV positive and coinfected with TB, who are likely to be receiving either the mechanism-based inhibitor of CYP3A, isoniazid, or the PXR agonist, rifampin, in addition to HAART.[71] Further confounding the issue is that PI-dependent proteosomal inhibition may also increase the expression of CYP2E1, leading to increased isoniazid hepatotoxicity.

Antiretroviral-associated portal hypertension is an important, new clinical condition. Patients often present with variceal bleeding, ascites, and other signs of decompensation. Prolonged exposure to didanosine may play a pathogenic role, and removal of the drug can result in clinical laboratory improvement.[72]

ANTIMICROBIAL AGENTS

Numerous antibiotics have been implicated in hepatotoxicity; however, hepatotoxicity is uncommon compared with other side effects such as gastrointestinal symptoms and allergic skin reactions. Even this infrequent incidence of acute severe liver injury has made antibiotic-induced liver injury a significant concern due to the frequency of antibiotic use. The US Food and Drug Administration closely monitors possible hepatotoxicity related to antibiotics and has affixed warning labels to several antibiotics currently on the market. Antibiotic-associated liver injury can present with various forms of acute and chronic liver injury rather than adhering to one specific pattern. DILI is a diagnosis of exclusion, and antimicrobial hepatotoxicity is often self-limited. Therefore, it is difficult to determine the true incidence of hepatotoxicity associated with antibiotic use. Data from a cohort study in France indicated that the crude incidence of drug-induced liver disease was 14 per 100,000 cases, with about 25% attributed to antibiotic use.[2] From a Spanish study, the estimated incidence of drug-induced hepatotoxicity was about 3.2 per 100,000 per year, and nearly one third of cases were attributed to antimicrobial agents.[73] Recent data from the NIH-sponsored Drug-Induced Liver Injury Network showed that 45% of cases in their database had antibiotic-induced hepatotoxicity.[74] Hepatotoxicity associated with antimicrobial use involves a spectrum of presentations including hepatocellular necrosis, hepatitis, cholestasis, steatosis, and granulomatous diseases. Most hepatotoxicity-related antimicrobial use is idiosyncratic; thus, it is difficult to evaluate mechanisms of injury in animal models. Several factors may play a role as secondary hits to increase susceptibility to hepatotoxicity, ranging from genetic variations in drug metabolizing activity to multiple medication use (see **Table 1**).

β-Lactams

An estimated incidence of heptatoxicity associated with amoxicillin and amoxicillin–clavulanic acid (amoxicillin–clavulanate; Augmentin) use is well documented, and is reported to be as high as 17 in 100,000 cases.[75] Amoxicillin is less frequently associated with hepatotoxicity. Hepatotoxicity is primarily related to clavulanic acid or its combination with amoxicillin. Hepatotoxicity occurs at variable times after administration of the drug, ranging from a few days to as much as 6 weeks. Cholestasis is the most common pattern of presentation of hepatotoxicity, and less frequently there is a combination of hepatocellular and cholestatic features. Other clinical features of hypersensitivity reactions such as skin rash, eosinophilia, and fever may be present indicating presumed immunologic idiosyncrasy as a mechanism of liver injury.[76] Hepatotoxicity associated with Augmentin use is usually mild and self-limited with abnormal liver enzymes resolving within 12 weeks. Prolonged use of Augmentin can cause chronic liver disease with cholestasis and ductopenia, although this is rare. The mechanism(s) of hepatotoxicity are still not completely clear; however, several human leukocyte antigen haplotypes have been found to be associated with hepatotoxicity, especially in elderly men.[77,78] Haplotype human leukocyte antigen (DRB1) seems to confer an increased risk of hepatotoxicity.[77,79] In a report from the Spanish registry, Augmentin was found to be the agent responsible for the highest number of cases of DILI.[73] Although there is liberal use of Augmentin worldwide, hepatotoxicity is uncommon, and acute severe liver injury is even rarer. However, the clinician should include it in the differential diagnosis of hepatotoxicity, and should closely observe the elderly male population. Amoxicillin is a rare cause of hepatotoxicity, and acute cholestasis has been reported.[80]

Ampicillin is rarely associated with hepatotoxicity, but a few case reports of Stevens-Johnson syndrome have been reported.[81] Ticarcillin, by itself, is not known to cause hepatotoxicity. Carbenicillin has caused hepatotoxicity in high doses,[82] the most common histologic pattern being a primary hepatocellular type of injury.

Semi-synthetic penicillinase-resistant compounds such as flucloxacillin, oxacillin, cloxacillin, and dicloxacillin are known to cause hepatotoxicity,[83,84] usually cholestatic hepatitis.[73,85] Flucloxacillin-induced hepatotoxicity may occasionally result in vanishing bile duct syndrome or biliary cirrhosis.[86] Onset of symptoms typically occurs 1 to 3 weeks after initiation of therapy and the exact mechanism(s) is unknown.

Cephalosporins rarely cause idiosyncratic hepatotoxicity.[87,88]

Macrolides

Macrolide antibiotics are a well-established cause of cholestatic type liver injury. Erythromycin estolate is the most common macrolide causing hepatotoxicity. However, other preparations of erythromycin, like propionate, ethylsuccinate, and stearate, can also cause hepatotoxicity.[89,90] The estimated risk of erythromycin-associated hepatotoxicity is approximately 3.6 cases per 100,000.[91] Symptoms usually occur 3 to 4 weeks after the initial course of therapy, and within 2 to 3 days during a subsequent course of erythromycin.[92] The mechanism of injury seems to be immunologic, and the pattern of injury is usually cholestatic. Nausea, vomiting, and abdominal pain may mimic acute cholecystitis. Infrequently, there is a skin rash and eosinophilia. Erythromycin-induced hepatotoxicity is usually reversible with drug discontinuation within 2 to 5 weeks, but rarely it may persist for 3 to 6 months. Erythromycin is not usually associated with severe fatal liver injury. In 2006, 3 reported cases of drug-induced hepatotoxicity were reported with telithromycin, one case requiring orthotopic liver transplantation and another resulting in death,[84] prompting a black box warning to be issued because of hepatotoxicity concerns.[85] Other macrolides like clarithromycin have also been associated with hepatotoxicity.

Fluoroquinolones

Ciprofloxacin, levofloxacin, ofloxacin, and norfloxacin have been reported to cause hepatotoxicity, but less frequently than other groups of antibiotics. Fluoroquinolones generally cause elevation in transaminases with minimal symptoms.[93] Fluoroquinolones have also been reported to cause severe liver injury requiring liver transplant. Ciprofloxacin is infrequently associated with significant hepatotoxicity, usually occurring within 3 weeks of exposure.[94,95] Trovafloxacin causes acute hepatitis as a result of immunologic idiosyncratic reaction, sometimes requiring liver transplant.[96,97] This problem resulted in withdrawal of trovafloxacin from the market. Fluoroquinolone-associated hepatotoxicity can result in hepatocellular and cholestatic acute liver injury, and even acute liver failure.

Tetracyclines

Tetracyclines are a well-recognized cause of hepatotoxicity, producing microvesicular steatosis.[98] High serum drug levels and female gender (especially pregnant women) are risk factors; children are less susceptible.[99] Renal impairment can increase serum levels due to reduced drug excretion, increasing the risk of hepatotoxicity. Within hepatocytes, the drug accumulates in mitochondria. Tetracyclines cause disruption of fatty acid oxidation and induce fat accumulation in liver. Tetracyclines such as oxytetracycline, chlortetracycline, minocycline, and demeclocycline can lead to dose-related microvesicular steatosis. Minocycline has been reported to cause hepatitis associated with hypersensitivity, which occurs within a few weeks of its use.[100] Prolonged use of minocycline in women can cause an autoimmune type reaction, presenting as a lupuslike syndrome in which autoimmune serologies including antinuclear antibody and anti–double stranded DNA antibody may be positive.[101] Rare cases of chronic cholestasis and vanishing bile duct syndrome have been reported secondary to tetracycline and doxycycline use.

Sulfonamides

Several sulfonamides such as sulfamethoxazole, trimethoprim–sulfamethoxazole (Bactrim or Septra), and sulfasalazine can cause hepatotoxicity; usually presenting as a hypersensitivity reaction occurring 5 to 14 days after starting treatment. Sometimes there is a reduced latency period after reintroduction of drug therapy, suggesting an immunoallergic component. The clinical presentation may involve multiple organ systems with lymphadenopathy, renal dysfunction, pancreatitis, and pulmonary lesions. Newer sulfonamides demonstrate fewer hypersensitivity reactions than older drugs. Patients with AIDS seem to be more susceptible to hypersensitivity reactions associated with sulfonamide use.[102] Genetic polymorphisms related to N-acetyltransferase enzyme activity play a role in susceptibility to liver injury; slow acetylators seem to be at higher risk for such hepatotoxicity.[103] Sulfonamide-associated hepatotoxicity is usually mild and reversible with a few weeks after discontinuation of drug therapy, however cholestasis may persist for 6 to 8 months. Occasionally, hepatotoxicity is severe and sometimes can be fatal. Cholestatic hepatitis with varying degrees of hepatocellular necrosis and bile duct injury are the usual findings on histology.[104]

Nitrofurantoin

Nitrofurantoin can have acute and chronic presentations, and can cause a wide variety of liver injury patterns including acute hepatocellular necrosis, cholestatic hepatitis, granulomas, chronic hepatitis, and even fibrosis and cirrhosis.[105–108] The acute form of liver injury is more common than the chronic type; however, nitrofurantoin rarely causes acute liver failure. Onset of acute cholestasis occurs after 6 weeks of treatment, whereas chronic hepatitis occurs after at least 6 months of nitrofurantoin use. Women are at higher risk for nitrofurantoin-induced liver injury. The estimated incidence of hepatotoxicity is around 3 to 20 per 1,000 cases.[109] A false positive antinuclear antibody and antismooth muscle antibody with nitrofurantoin-associated chronic hepatitis suggest an immunoallergic type of liver injury;[109] however, cell mediated mechanisms may also play a role.[110] Rechallenge with nitrofurantoin should not be attempted. Cross-sensitivity with other furan derivatives, such as furosemide and furazolidone, has been reported.[111]

Antifungal Agents

With the exception of some instances of abnormal liver enzyme tests, antifungal agents are not frequently associated with hepatotoxicity. Antifungals such as itraconazole, flucytosine, and terbinafine are more commonly associated with hepatotoxicity than amphotericin B. Ketoconazole is the most common antifungal associated with liver injury. Some recommend measuring liver tests periodically if patients are on a prolonged course of antifungal treatment.[112] Hepatotoxicity is usually self-limited after drug discontinuation.

Antituberculous Agents

Antituberculous agents are associated with a wide range of side effects involving multiple organs. However, hepatotoxicity is frequent and often serious. Hepatotoxicity caused by a specific antituberculous agent is often difficult to identify because the drugs are generally used in combination regimens. Aside from streptomycin, most common antituberculous medications have been associated with hepatotoxicity.

Isoniazid

Isoniazid is a synthetic bactericidal antibiotic that has been used to treat *Mycobacterium tuberculosis* for more than 50 years.[9] Isoniazid is the antimicrobial agent most frequently cited in cases of drug-induced hepatotoxicity worldwide, in terms of both overall number of cases and rate of cases per exposure to the drug, and this is due, in part, to its extensive use. Drug-induced hepatotoxicity caused by isoniazid is characterized by hepatocellular necrosis, which in some cases can progress to liver failure and death.[113] Liver injury from isoniazid seems to be mediated by the toxic metabolite hydrazine and its monoacetyl derivative.[9] Most increased aminotransferase levels appear within several weeks following initiation of treatment. Ten to twenty percent of patients taking isoniazid will develop this modest elevation in aminotransaminases without development of signs or symptoms suggestive of liver disease. In many of these patients, continuation of isoniazid is well tolerated and their aminotransferase levels will return to normal or nearly normal levels, representing a hepatic adaptation response (see Acetaminophen section).[9,113,114] An estimated 0.1% to 2.0% of patients treated with isoniazid will develop significant clinical hepatitis.[9,113] Combination of isoniazid with other antituberculin drugs including rifampin and pyrazinamide increases the likelihood of toxicity with isoniazid.[12,114] In a metaanalysis by Steele and colleagues,[115] the incidence of clinical hepatitis with isoniazid alone was found to be 0.6%. Isoniazid in a combination of drugs without rifampin causes clinical hepatitis 1.6% of the time. Combination antituberculous therapy with rifampin but without isoniazid has a 1.1% incidence of clinical hepatitis, and when isoniazid and rifampin regimens are used together, there is a 2.5% incidence of clinical hepatitis.[115] Rifapmin is a well-characterized ligand for the PXR and induces the expression of several drug metabolizing enzymes, most notably CYP3A, which can alter the metabolism and potential hepatotoxicity of a large number of drugs, including isoniazid.[115] Another important consideration is that the metabolism of isoniazid depends on the genotype of the *N*-acetyltransferase 2 allelle. Thus, patients can have different rates of isoniazid acetylation, the major route of metabolism, with slow acetylators being more susceptible to isoniazid-dependent liver injury.[116,117]

Rifampin

Hepatotoxicity associated with rifampin use is less frequent than with isoniazid use. The usual histologic pattern is cholestasis, likely because rifampin is a competitive inhibitor of bile salt uptake and bile salt export. Rifampin is sometimes associated with hypersensitivity type reactions.[118] Affected individuals, however, are usually asymptomatic and rarely recognized clinically.

Pyrazinamide

An antituberculous regimen with pyrazinamide is more commonly associated with hepatotoxicity when given with rifampin or isoniazid. Occasionally, pyrazinamide has been noted to cause dose-dependent hepatotoxicity. Although the mechanism of hepatotoxicity has been considered to be dose-related, in one case report rechallenge after an initial reaction to a combination regimen led to an intense elevation in serum aminotransferase levels with eosinophilia, suggesting a hypersensitivity reaction.[119]

ACETAMINOPHEN

Acetaminophen hepatotoxicity represents a classic form of direct toxicity and likely adaptation to hepatotoxicity. Acetaminophen is a widely used nonprescription analgesic and antipyretic agent. It is also a dose-related hepatotoxin and the leading cause of acute liver failure in the United States. Acetaminophen-induced hepatotoxicity can occur with massive overdoses or with therapeutic doses in certain susceptible individuals. This liver injury is due not to the drug itself but to the formation of the toxic metabolite, *N*-acetyl-*p*-benzoquinine imine, generated through the cytochrome P450 drug-metabolizing system. Normally, hepatic stores of glutathione combine with the toxic metabolite and prevent liver cell injury. When glutathione stores are depleted, the excess metabolite binds to liver cell proteins causing hepatic cell death. CYP2E1 is induced by alcohol consumption and possibly starvation, as is glutathione depletion. Hence, regular consumption of alcohol or starvation may make a person more susceptible to this form of hepatotoxicity. Despite our already detailed understanding of acetaminophen hepatotoxicity, new information is emerging. Proinflammatory cytokines/chemokines and the innate immune system are increasingly recognized as playing critical roles in acetaminophen-induced liver injury.[120] Clinically, our ability to diagnose acetaminophen toxicity in questionable cases, especially those who arrive at the emergency room long after their overdose and when blood levels are undetectable,[121] may be enhanced by new assays to detect acetaminophen–protein adducts. Moreover, in recent studies of human volunteers given 4 g of acetaminophen in a daily dose (the upper recommended dose), increased liver enzymes were frequently seen immediately after initiating acetaminophen therapy.[122] Subjects were initially tested daily, which may explain this observation. Acetaminophen is likely one of a series of drugs that induces liver injury initially, but then the liver adapts to this toxic response and liver enzymes normalize with continued therapy. An example of this adaptive pathway is the Keap1-Nrf2 antioxidant defense system.[123] Disruption of this system sensitizes to acetaminophen-induced hepatotoxicity. A variety of nutritional and environmental factors can enhance and disrupt these adaptive pathways. Thus, several forms of liver injury, including isoniazid, statins, and acetaminophen, likely induce initial low-grade hepatotoxicity that will resolve over time with induction of defense systems. Inability to appropriately activate these defense systems due to genetic or environmental factors may play a critical role in the development of hepatotoxicity.[124]

COMPLEMENTARY AND ALTERNATIVE MEDICINE (CAM)

Complementary and alternative medicines are widely used and patients frequently do not inform their physicians about their CAM use.[125] The safety of CAM agents is not well established, in large part because of a lack of regulatory guidelines. In 1994, Congress passed the Dietary Supplement Health and Education Act, which exempted dietary supplement producers from many Food and Drug Administration regulations.

Table 2
CAM agents/nutritional supplements and form of hepatotoxicity

Herb	Type of Liver Injury
Crotalaria Heliotropium Senecio longilobus Symphytum officinale (pyrrolizidine alkaloids)	Sinusoidal obstruction syndrome (veno-occlusive disease)
Chaparral leaf, germander	Zone 3 necrosis, cirrhosis, cholestasis, chronic hepatitis
Pennyroyal (squamit) oil	Zone 3 necrosis, microvesicular steatosis, fulminant liver failure
Jin Bu Huan	Acute and chronic cholestatic hepatitis, microvesicular steatosis, fibrosis
Mistletoe	Chronic hepatitis
Margosa oil	Microvesicular steatosis, Reye syndrome, hepatic necrosis
Usnic acid	Fulminant liver failure
Atractylis gummifera	Acute hepatitis, fulminant liver failure
Callilepis laureola	Acute hepatitis, fulminant liver failure
Impila	Acute hepatitis, fulminant liver failure
Camphor	Necrolytic hepatitis
Cascara sagrada	Cholestatic hepatitis
TJ-8, Dai saiko-toi	Autoimmune hepatitis
TJ-9, Sho-saiko-to	Acute and chronic hepatitis
Paeonia spp.	Acute hepatitis, fulminant liver failure
Greater celandine	Chronic hepatitis, cholestasis, fibrosis
Germander	Acute and chronic hepatitis, fulminant liver failure
Isabgol	Giant cell hepatitis
Kava	Acute and chronic hepatitis, fulminant liver failure
Ma Huang	Acute hepatitis, autoimmune hepatitis
Oil of cloves	Hepatic necrosis
Sassafras	Hepatocarcinogen
Saw palmetto	Mild hepatitis
Shou-wu-pian	Acute hepatitis
Valerian	Mild hepatitis

Concerns about safety relate to product content, direct toxicity, and CAM–drug interactions. There is great variability in the composition of herbal products/supplements, with some products containing only a small fraction of the advertised dose.[126–128] This product variability is probably an unavoidable aspect of many Chinese herbal compounds. Some CAM products are contaminated with drugs/toxins. Moreover, some Chinese patent medicines deliberately contain small amounts of prescription drugs (eg, antibiotics, ephedrine, methyltestosterone).[126,129] These drugs may also be contaminated with heavy metals (eg, lead, arsenic, mercury).[130] Toxicity induced by CAM products is well described.[127,131] Hepatotoxicity is one of the most frequently reported side effects of CAM products (eg, germander and pyrrolizidine alkaloid–containing compounds), sometimes leading to potentially fatal liver failure.[131–133] Recently reported cases of hepatotoxicity due to kava kava and to various weight loss agents have heightened awareness of this problem and have reinforced the need to carefully question patients with elevated liver enzymes about CAM use (**Table 2** gives examples of CAM hepatotoxicity).[134] A recent report highlighted the risk of fulminant hepatic failure requiring liver transplantation due to CAM ingestion.[135] CAM agents can interact adversely with traditional medications. An example is the potential interactions of St John's wort with cyclosporine and indinavir.[136] This interaction was highlighted when cardiac transplant patients underwent rejection shortly after starting St John's wort, presumably because of the induction of CYP3A4 by the St John's wort.[137] Because of the potential for toxicity–drug interactions, the patient and health care provider need to be optimally educated about CAM. The Physicians' Desk Reference for Herbal Medicines and the Physicians' Desk Reference for Nutritional Supplements, the Web sites of the Cochrane Database System Reviews (http://www.cochrane.org), and the NCCAM (http://nccam.nih.gov) are valuable sources for updated information.

SUMMARY

Drug-induced hepatotoxicity is a rare but important complication that will continue to be problematic with new drugs coming on to the market. Initial clinical trials are not always adequately powered to determine which medications are hepatotoxic. It is the health care system's, including the physician's, responsibility to monitor and report drug-induced hepatotoxicity. Recent studies reinforce the important role of antibiotics in causing hepatotoxicity; the relative safety of statins, reinforcing the lack of need for regular liver enzyme monitoring; the importance of acetaminophen in fulminant liver failure; and the need to remain cognizant of CAM hepatotoxicity. A systematic approach should be taken to determine the cause of hepatotoxicity and remove the offending agent. A thorough history is essential and should be correlated with the pattern of liver test abnormality, latency of symptom onset, and presence or absence of immune hypersensitivity.

REFERENCES

1. Lee WM. Drug-induced hepatotoxicity. N Engl J Med 2003;349(5):474–85.
2. Sgro C, Clinard F, Ouazir K, et al. Incidence of drug-induced hepatic injuries: a French population-based study. Hepatology 2002;36(2):451–5.
3. Nathwani RA, Kaplowitz N. Drug hepatotoxicity. Clin Liver Dis 2006;10(2): 207–17, vii.
4. Chang CY, Schiano TD. Review article: drug hepatotoxicity. Aliment Pharmacol Ther 2007;25(10):1135–51.

5. Fontana RJ. Acute liver failure including acetaminophen overdose. Med Clin North Am 2008;92(4):761–94, viii.

6. Wilkinson GR. Drug metabolism and variability among patients in drug response. N Engl J Med 2005;352(21):2211–21.

7. Gunawan BK, Kaplowitz N. Mechanisms of drug-induced liver disease. Clin Liver Dis 2007;11(3):459–75, v.

8. Sotaniemi EA, Arranto AJ, Pelkonen O, et al. Age and cytochrome P450-linked drug metabolism in humans: an analysis of 226 subjects with equal histopathologic conditions. Clin Pharmacol Ther 1997;61(3):331–9.

9. Maddrey WC. Drug-induced hepatotoxicity: 2005. J Clin Gastroenterol 2005;39(4 Suppl 2):S83–9.

10. Castell JV, Castell M. Allergic hepatitis induced by drugs. Curr Opin Allergy Clin Immunol 2006;6(4):258–65.

11. Lewis JH. Medication-related and other forms of toxic liver injury. In: Brandt LJ, editor. Clinical practice of gastroenterology. Philadelphia: Churchill Livingstone; 1998. p. 855.

12. Lee WM. Drug-induced hepatotoxicity. N Engl J Med 1995;333(17):1118–27.

13. Lee WM, Seremba E. Etiologies of acute liver failure. Curr Opin Crit Care 2008;14(2):198–201.

14. Toth PP, Davidson MH. High-dose statin therapy: benefits and safety in aggressive lipid lowering. J Fam Pract 2008;57(5 Suppl High-Dose):S29–36.

15. Bhardwaj SS, Chalasani N. Lipid-lowering agents that cause drug-induced hepatotoxicity. Clin Liver Dis 2007;11(3):597–613, vii.

16. Cohen DE, Anania FA, Chalasani N. An assessment of statin safety by hepatologists. Am J Cardiol 2006;97(8A):77C–81C.

17. Anfossi G, Massucco P, Bonomo K, et al. Prescription of statins to dyslipidemic patients affected by liver diseases: a subtle balance between risks and benefits. Nutr Metab Cardiovasc Dis 2004;14(4):215–24.

18. Marino G, Lewis JH. Drug-induced liver disease. Curr Opin Gastroenterol 2001;17(3):232–41.

19. Bristol-Myers Squibb. Product information. Pravachol [pravastatin]. Princeton (NJ): Bristol-Myers Squibb Company; 2007.

20. Tolman KG. Defining patient risks from expanded preventive therapies. Am J Cardiol 2000;85(12A):15E–9E.

21. Merck/Schering-Plough. Product information. Zetia [Ezetimibe]. North Wales (PA): Merck/Schering-Plough Pharmaceuticals; 2007.

22. Tuteja S, Pyrsopoulos NT, Wolowich WR, et al. Simvastatin-ezetimibe-induced hepatic failure necessitating liver transplantation. Pharmacotherapy 2008;28(9):1188–93.

23. Pieper JA. Overview of niacin formulations: differences in pharmacokinetics, efficacy, and safety. Am J Health Syst Pharm 2003;60(13 Suppl 2):S9–14, quiz S25.

24. McCormack PL, Keating GM. Prolonged-release nicotinic acid: a review of its use in the treatment of dyslipidaemia. Drugs 2005;65(18):2719–40.

25. Dalton TA, Berry RS. Hepatotoxicity associated with sustained-release niacin. Am J Med 1992;93(1):102–4.

26. Madariaga MG. Drug-related hepatotoxicity. N Engl J Med 2006;354(20):2191–3 [author reply 2191–3].

27. Patel SD, Taylor HC. Intrahepatic cholestasis during nicotinic acid therapy. Cleve Clin J Med 1994;61(1):70–5, quiz 80–2.

28. Clementz GL, Holmes AW. Nicotinic acid-induced fulminant hepatic failure. J Clin Gastroenterol 1987;9(5):582–4.

29. Mullin GE, Greenson JK, Mitchell MC. Fulminant hepatic failure after ingestion of sustained-release nicotinic acid. Ann Intern Med 1989;111(3):253–5.

30. Hodis HN. Acute hepatic failure associated with the use of low-dose sustained-release niacin. JAMA 1990;264(2):181.

31. McKenney J. New perspectives on the use of niacin in the treatment of lipid disorders. Arch Intern Med 2004;164(7):697–705.

32. McKenney JM, Proctor JD, Harris S, et al. A comparison of the efficacy and toxic effects of sustained- vs immediate-release niacin in hypercholesterolemic patients. JAMA 1994;271(9):672–7.

33. Lucena MI, Andrade RJ, Vicioso L, et al. Prolonged cholestasis after raloxifene and fenofibrate interaction: a case report. World J Gastroenterol 2006;12(32): 5244–6.

34. de Diego Lorenzo A, Catalina V, Garcia Sanchez A, et al. [Cholestatic hepatitis caused by gemfibrozil]. Rev Esp Enferm Dig 2001;93(9):610–1.

35. Graham DJ, Green L, Senior JR, et al. Troglitazone-induced liver failure: a case study. Am J Med 2003;114:299–306.

36. Chan KA, Truman A, Gurwitz JH, et al. A cohort study of the incidence of serious acute liver injury in diabetic patients treated with hypoglycemic agents. Arch Intern Med 2003;163(6):728–34.

37. Marcy TR, Britton ML, Blevins SM. Second-generation thiazolidinediones and hepatotoxicity. Ann Pharmacother 2004;38:1419–23.

38. Forman LM, Simmons DA, Diamond RH. Hepatic failure in a patient taking rosiglitazone. Ann Intern Med 2000;132(2):118–21.

39. Al-Salman J, Arjomand H, Kemp DG, et al. Hepatocellular injury in a patient receiving rosiglitazone. A case report. Ann Intern Med 2000;132:121–4.

40. Farley-Hills E, Sivasankar R, Martin M. Fatal liver failure associated with pioglitazone. BMJ 2004;329(7463):429.

41. Chase MP, Yarze JC. Pioglitazone-associated fulminant hepatic failure. Am J Gastroenterol 2002;97:502–3.

42. GlaxoSmithKline. Product information: Avandia [Rosiglitazone]. Research Triangle Park (NC): GlaxoSmithKline; April 2007.

43. Takeda Pharmaceuticals. Product information: Actos [Pioglitazone]. Deerfield (IL): Takeda Pharmaceuticals America, Inc; August 2007.

44. DeSanty KP. Antidepressant-induced liver injury. Ann Pharmacother 2007;41(7): 1201–11.

45. GlaxoSmithKline. Product information: Paxil [paroxetine]. Research Triangle Park (NC): GlaxoSmithKline; January 2008.

46. Bristol-Myers Squibb. Product information: Serzone [Nefazodone]. Princeton (NJ): Bristol-Myers Squibb Company; October 2003.

47. Watkins P. COMT inhibitors and liver toxicity. Neurology 2000;55(11):S51–2.

48. Lew MF, Kricorian G. Results from a 2-year centralized tolcapone liver enzyme monitoring program. Clin Neuropharmacol 2007;30:281–6.

49. Valeant Pharmaceuticals. Product information: Tasmar [Tolcapone]. Costa Mesa (CA): Valeant Pharmaceuticals International; December 2006.

50. Temesgen Z, Wright AJ. Antiretrovirals. Mayo Clin Proc 1999;74(12):1284–301.

51. Vogel M, Rockstroh JK. Hepatotoxicity and liver disease in the context of HIV therapy. Curr Opin HIV AIDS 2007;2(4):306–13.

52. Sulkowski MS, Thomas DL, Chaisson RE, et al. Hepatotoxicity associated with antiretroviral therapy in adults infected with human immunodeficiency virus and the role of hepatitis C or B virus infection. JAMA 2000;283(1):74–80.

53. Nuñez M. Hepatotoxicity of antiretrovirals: incidence, mechanisms and management. J Hepatol 2006;44(Suppl 1):S132–9.
54. Nuñez M, Soriano V. Hepatotoxicity of antiretrovirals: incidence, mechanisms and management. Drug Saf 2005;28(1):53–66.
55. Johnson A, Ray A, Hanes J, et al. Toxicity of antiviral nucleoside analogs and the human mitochondrial DNA polymerase. J Biol Chem 2001;276:40847–57.
56. Parker RA, Flint OP, Mulvey R, et al. Endoplasmic reticulum stress links dyslipidemia to inhibition of proteosome activity and glucose transport by HIV protease inhibitors. Mol Pharmacol 2005;67(6):1909–19.
57. Cooper CL. HIV antiretroviral medications and hepatotoxicity. Curr Opin HIV AIDS 2007;2(6):466–73.
58. Lai KK, Gang DL, Zawacki JK, et al. Fulminant hepatic failure associated with 2′, 3′-dideoxyinosine (ddI). Ann Intern Med 1991;115:283–4.
59. Bristol-Myers Squibb. Product information: Videx EC [didanosine]. Princeton (NJ): Bristol-Myers Squibb Company; March 2007.
60. Bristol-Myers Squibb. Product information: Zerit [stavudine]. Princeton (NJ): Bristol-Myers Squibb Company; July 2008.
61. Boehringer Ingelheim Pharmaceuticals. Product information: Viramune [nevirapine]. Ridgefield (CT): Boehringer Ingelheim Pharmaceuticals, Inc.; June 2008.
62. Boehringer Ingelheim Pharmaceuticals. Product information: Aptivus [tipranavir]. Ridgefield (CT): Boehringer Ingelheim Pharmaceuticals, Inc.; 2008.
63. Hurst M, Noble S. Stavudine: an update of its use in the treatment of HIV infection. Drugs 1999;58(5):919–49.
64. Abbott Laboratories. Product information: Norvir [ritonavir]. North Chicago: Abbott Laboratories; May 2007.
65. Jain MK. Drug-induced liver injury associated with HIV medications. Clin Liver Dis 2007;11(3):615–39.
66. Cooper CL, Parbhakar MA, Angel JB. Hepatotoxicity associated with antiretroviral therapy containing dual versus single protease inhibitors in individuals coinfected with hepatitis C virus and human immunodeficiency virus. Clin Infect Dis 2002;34(9):1259–63.
67. Piccinini M, Rinaudo MT, Chiapello N, et al. The human 26S proteasome is a target of antiretroviral agents. AIDS 2002;16(5):693–700.
68. Riddle TM, Kuhel DG, Woollett LA, et al. HIV protease inhibitor induces fatty acid and sterol biosynthesis in liver and adipose tissues due to the accumulation of activated sterol regulatory element-binding proteins in the nucleus. J Biol Chem 2001;276(40):37514–9. Epub 2001 Aug 23.
69. King J, Wynn H, Brundage R, et al. Pharmacokinetic enhancement of protease inhibitor therapy. Clin Pharm 2004;43(5):291–310.
70. Slain D, Pakyz A, Israel D, et al. Variability in activity of hepatic CYP3A4 in patients infected with HIV. Pharmacotherapy 2000;20:898–907.
71. Wen X, Wang JS, Neuvonen PJ, Backman JT. Isoniazid is a mechanism-based inhibitor of cytochrome P450 1A2, 2A6, 2C19 and 3A4 isoforms in human liver microsomes. Eur J Clin Pharmacol 2002;57:799–804.
72. Maida I, Garcia-Gasco P, Sotgiu G, et al. Antiretroviral-associated portal hypertension: a new clinical condition? Prevalence, predictors and outcome. Antivir Ther 2008;13(1):103–7.
73. Andrade RJ, Lucena MI, Fernandez MC, et al. Drug-induced liver injury: an analysis of 461 incidences submitted to the Spanish registry over a 10-year period. Gastroenterology 2005;129:512–21.

74. Chalasani N, Fontana RJ, Bonkovsky HL, et al. Drug Induced Liver Injury Network (DILIN). Causes, clinical features, and outcomes from a prospective study of drug-induced liver injury in the United States. Gastroenterology 2008; 135(6):1924–34, 1934.e1-4. Epub 2008 Sep 17.

75. Garcia Rodriguez LA, Stricker BH, Zimmerman HJ. Risk of acute liver injury associated with the combination of amoxicillin and clavulanic acid. Arch Intern Med 1996;156:1327–32.

76. Mari JY, Guy C, Beyens MN, et al. [Delayed drug-induced hepatic injury. Evoking the role of amoxicillin-clavulinic acid combination]. Therapie 2000;55:699–704.

77. O'Donohue J, Oien KA, Donaldson P, et al. Co-amoxiclav jaundice: clinical and histological features and HLA class II association. Gut 2000;47:717–20.

78. Gresser U. Amoxicillin-clavulanic acid therapy may be associated with severe side effects—review of the literature. Eur J Med Res 2001;6:139–49.

79. Hautekeete ML, Horsmans Y, Van Waeyenberge C, et al. HLA association of amoxicillin-clavulanate–induced hepatitis. Gastroenterology 1999;117:1181–6.

80. Bolzan H, Spatola J, Castelletto R, et al. [Intrahepatic cholestasis induced by amoxicillin alone]. Gastroenterol Hepatol 2000;23:237–9.

81. Beard K, Belic L, Aselton P, et al. Outpatient drug-induced parenchymal liver disease requiring hospitalization. J Clin Pharmacol 1986;26:633–7.

82. Wilson FM, Belamaric J, Lauter CB, et al. Anicteric carbenicillin hepatitis. Eight episodes in four patients. JAMA 1975;232:818–21.

83. Goldstein LI, Granoff M, Waisman J. Hepatic injury due to oxacillin administration. Am J Gastroenterol 1978;70:171–4.

84. Pollock AA, Berger SA, Simberkoff MS, et al. Hepatitis associated with high-dose oxacillin therapy. Arch Intern Med 1978;138:915–7.

85. De Valle MB, Av Klinteberg V, Alem N, et al. Drug-induced liver injury in a Swedish University hospital out-patient hepatology clinic. Aliment Pharmacol Ther 2006;24:1187–95.

86. Davies MH, Harrison RF, Elias E, et al. Antibiotic-associated acute vanishing bile duct syndrome: a pattern associated with severe, prolonged, intrahepatic cholestasis. J Hepatol 1994;20:112–6.

87. Eggleston SM, Belandres MM. Jaundice associated with cephalosporin therapy. Drug Intell Clin Pharm 1985;19:553–5.

88. Ammann R, Neftel K, Hardmeier T, et al. Cephalosporin-induced cholestatic jaundice. Lancet 1982;2:336–7.

89. Horn S, Aglas F, Horina JH. Cholestasis and liver cell damage due to hypersensitivity to erythromycin stearate – recurrence following therapy with erythromycin succinate. Wien Klin Wochenschr 1999;111:76–7.

90. Keeffe EB, Reis TC, Berland JE. Hepatotoxicity to both erythromycin estolate and erythromycin ethylsuccinate. Dig Dis Sci 1982;27:701–4.

91. Derby LE, Jick H, Henry DA, et al. Erythromycin-associated cholestatic hepatitis. Med J Aust 1993;158:600–2.

92. Braun P. Hepatotoxicity of erythromycin. J Infect Dis 1969;119:300–6.

93. Ball P, Mandell L, Niki Y, et al. Comparative tolerability of the newer fluoroquinolone antibacterials. Drug Saf 1999;21:407–21.

94. Villeneuve JP, Davies C, Cote J. Suspected ciprofloxacin-induced hepatotoxicity. Ann Pharmacother 1995;29:257–9.

95. Grassmick BK, Lehr VT, Sundareson AS. Fulminant hepatic failure possibly related to ciprofloxacin. Ann Pharmacother 1992;26:636–9.

96. Chen HJ, Bloch KJ, Maclean JA. Acute eosinophilic hepatitis from trovafloxacin. N Engl J Med 2000;342:359–60.

97. Lucena MI, Andrade RJ, Rodrigo L, et al. Trovafloxacin-induced acute hepatitis. Clin Infect Dis 2000;30:400–1.
98. Dowling HF, Lepper MH. Hepatic reactions to tetracycline. JAMA 1964;188:307–9.
99. Whalley PJ, Adams RH, Combes B. Tetracycline toxicity in pregnancy. Liver and pancreatic dysfunction. JAMA 1964;189:357–62.
100. Lawrenson RA, Seaman HE, Sundstrom A, et al. Liver damage associated with minocycline use in acne: a systematic review of the published literature and pharmacovigilance data. Drug Saf 2000;23:333–49.
101. Bhat G, Jordan J Jr, Sokalski S, et al. Minocycline-induced hepatitis with auto-immune features and neutropenia. J Clin Gastroenterol 1998;27:74–5.
102. Gordin FM, Simon GL, Wofsy CB, et al. Adverse reactions to trimethoprim-sulfa-methoxazole in patients with the acquired immunodeficiency syndrome. Ann Intern Med 1984;100:495–9.
103. Rieder MJ. Mechanisms of unpredictable adverse drug reactions. Drug Saf 1994;11:196–212.
104. Fries J, Siragenian R. Sulfonamide hepatitis. Report of a case due to sulfame-thoxazole and sulfisoxazole. N Engl J Med 1966;274:95–7.
105. Young TL, Achkar E, Tuthill R, et al. Chronic active hepatitis induced by nitrofur-antoin. Cleve Clin Q 1985;52:253–6.
106. Berry WR, Warren GH, Reichen J. Nitrofurantoin-induced cholestatic hepatitis from cow's milk in a teenaged boy. West J Med 1984;140:278–80.
107. Sharp JR, Ishak KG, Zimmerman HJ. Chronic active hepatitis and severe hepatic necrosis associated with nitrofurantoin. Ann Intern Med 1980;92:14–9.
108. Strohscheer H, Wegener HH. [Nitrofurantoin-induced granulomatous hepatitis]. MMW Munch Med Wochenschr 1977;119:1535–6.
109. Stricker BH, Blok AP, Claas FH, et al. Hepatic injury associated with the use of nitrofurans: a clinicopathological study of 52 reported cases. Hepatology 1988;8:599–606.
110. Kelly BD, Heneghan MA, Bennani F, et al. Nitrofurantoin-induced hepatotoxicity mediated by CD8+ T cells. Am J Gastroenterol 1998;93:819–21.
111. Engel JJ, Vogt TR, Wilson DE. Cholestatic hepatitis after administration of furan derivatives. Arch Intern Med 1975;135:733–5.
112. Franks AL, Binkin NJ, Snider DE Jr, et al. Isoniazid hepatitis among pregnant and postpartum Hispanic patients. Public Health Rep 1989;104:151–5.
113. Polson JE. Hepatotoxicity due to antibiotics. Clin Liver Dis 2007;11(3):549–61.
114. Senior JR. Drug hepatotoxicity from a regulatory perspective. Clin Liver Dis 2007;11(3):507–24.
115. Steele M, Burk R, DesPrez R. Toxic hepatitis with isoniazid and rifampin. A meta-analysis. Chest 1991;99:465–71.
116. Lehmann J, McKee D, Watson MA, et al. The human orphan nuclear receptor PXR is activated by compounds that regulate CYP3A4 gene expression and cause drug interactions. J Clin Invest 1998;102:1016–23.
117. Dickinson DS, Bailey WC, Hirschowitz BI, et al. Risk factors for isoniazid (NIH)-induced liver dysfunction. J Clin Gastroenterol 1981;3:271–9.
118. Huang Y-S, Chern H-D, Su W-J, et al. Polymorphism of the N-acetyltransferase 2 gene as a susceptibility risk factor for antituberculosis drug-induced hepatitis. Hepatology 2002;35:883–9.
119. Saukkonen JJ, Cohn DL, Jasmer RM, et al. An official ATS statement: hepato-toxicity of antituberculosis therapy. Am J Respir Crit Care Med 2006;174:935–52.

120. Masubuchi Y, Sugiyama S, Horie T. Th1/Th2 cytokine balance as a determinant of acetaminophen-induced liver injury. Chem Biol Interact 2008 [Epub ahead of print].

121. James LP, Capparelli EV, Simpson PM, et al. Network of Pediatric Pharmacology Research Units, National Institutes of Child Health and Human Development. Acetaminophen-associated hepatic injury: evaluation of acetaminophen protein adducts in children and adolescents with acetaminophen overdose. Clin Pharmacol Ther 2008;84(6):684–90.

122. Watkins PB, Kaplowitz N, Slattery JT, et al. Aminotransferase elevations in healthy adults receiving 4 grams of acetaminophen daily: a randomized controlled trial. JAMA 2006;296(1):87–93.

123. Copple IM, Goldring CE, Kitteringham NR, et al. The Nrf2-Keap1 defence pathway: role in protection against drug-induced toxicity. Toxicology 2008; 246(1):24–33. Epub 2007 Nov 12.

124. McClain CJ, Price S, Barve S, et al. Acetaminophen hepatotoxicity: an update. Curr Gastroenterol Rep 1999;1(1):42–9.

125. McClain CJ, Dryden G, Krueger K. Complementary and alternative medicine in gastroenterology. In: Yamada T, editor. Textbook of gastroenterology, 5th edition. Wiley-Blackwell; 2008. p. 2844–59.

126. Angell M, Kassirer JP. Alternative medicine—the risks of untested and unregulated remedies. N Engl J Med 1998;339(12):839–41.

127. Shaw D, Leon C, Koley S, et al. Traditional remedies and food supplements. A 5-year toxicological study (1991–1995). Drug Saf 1997;17(5):342–56.

128. Cui J, Garle M, Eneroin P, et al. What do commercial ginseng preparations contain? Lancet 1994;344:134.

129. Ko RJ. Adulterants in Asian patent medicines. N Engl J Med 1998;339:847.

130. Beigel Y, Ostfeld I, Schoenfeld N. Clinical problem-solving. A leading question. N Engl J Med 1998;339(12):827–30.

131. Schuppan D, Jia JD, Brinkhavs R, et al. Herbal products for liver diseases: a therapeutic challenge for the new millennium. Hepatology 1999;30(4): 1099–104.

132. Kaplowitz N. Hepatotoxicity of herbal remedies: insights into the intricacies of plant-animal warfare and cell death. Gastroenterology 1997;113(4):1408–12.

133. Lekehal M, Pessayre D, Lereau JM, et al. Hepatotoxicity of the herbal medicine germander: metabolic activation of its furano diterpenoids by cytochrome P450 3A depletes cytoskeleton-associated protein thiols and forms plasma membrane blebs in rat hepatocytes. Hepatology 1996;24(1):212–8.

134. Hanje AJ, Fortune B, Song M, et al. The use of selected nutritional supplements and complementary and alternative medicine in liver disease. Nutr Clin Pract 2006;21:255–72.

135. Estes JD, Stolpman D, Olyaei A, et al. High prevalence of potentially hepatotoxic herbal supplement use in patients with fulminant hepatic failure. Arch Surg 2003;138:852–8.

136. Ruschitzka F, Meier PJ, Turina M, et al. Acute heart transplant rejection due to Saint John's wort. Lancet 2000;355(9203):548–9.

137. Piscitelli SC, Burstein AH, Chaitt D, et al. Indinavir concentrations and St. John's wort. Lancet 2000;355(9203):547–8.

Management of Autoimmune and Cholestatic Liver Disorders

Karen L. Krok, MD[a], Santiago J. Munoz, MD, FACP, FACG[b,c],*

KEYWORDS

- Autoimmune hepatitis • Biliary cirrhosis
- Sclerosing cholangitis • Overlap syndrome
- Cholestasis • Liver transplantation

The management of autoimmune and cholestatic liver disorders is a challenging area of hepatology. Autoimmune and cholestatic liver diseases represent a comparatively small proportion of hepatobiliary disorders, yet their appropriate management is of critical importance for patient survival. In this article, management strategies are discussed, including the indications and expectations of pharmacologic therapy, endoscopic approaches, and the role of liver transplantation.

AUTOIMMUNE HEPATITIS

Autoimmune hepatitis is an inflammatory liver disease of unknown cause. The disease can present with the onset of jaundice and marked elevation of amino liver transaminases. In some patients, autoimmune hepatitis may present as symptomatic, chronically elevated liver enzymes, or incidentally found cryptogenic cirrhosis, or more rarely, as acute fulminant liver failure.[1–4] Patients with autoimmune hepatitis typically have circulating autoantibodies at robust titers, elevated globulins, plasma cells, lymphocytic inflammation and periportal liver cell necrosis on hepatic histology.[1,5] An immune mediated injury in genetically susceptible persons, perhaps triggered or modulated by environmental agents, is believed to lead to liver damage in

[a] Division of Gastroenterology and Hepatology, University of Pennsylvania School of Medicine, 3400 Spruce Street, 3 Ravdin, Philadelphia, PA 19104, USA
[b] Temple School of Medicine, 3322 North Broad Street, Philadelphia, PA 19140, USA
[c] Temple University Hospital, 3322 North Broad Street, Suite 148, Medical Office Building, Philadelphia, PA 19140, USA
* Corresponding author. Temple University Hospital, Liver Transplant Program, 3322 North Broad Street, Suite 148, Philadelphia, PA 19140.
E-mail address: Santiago.Munoz@tuhs.temple.edu (S.J. Munoz).

Clin Liver Dis 13 (2009) 295–316
doi:10.1016/j.cld.2009.02.011
1089-3261/09/$ – see front matter © 2009 Elsevier Inc. All rights reserved.

liver.theclinics.com

autoimmune hepatitis.[6–8] The syndrome, diagnosis, and natural history of autoimmune hepatitis have been reviewed in detail elsewhere.[1,2,9,10]

Management

In general, management strategies in patients with autoimmune hepatitis are individualized and tailored to the clinical, biochemical, and histologic severity. The classic presentation, with jaundice, systemic symptoms, marked elevation of alanine aminotransferase (ALT), aspartate aminotransferase, and elevated globulins in a young or middle aged woman, is typically treated with corticosteroids, or a combination of high doses of corticosteroids and antimetabolites (see later discussion). In contrast, autoimmune hepatitis presenting with acute liver failure may require urgent liver transplantation. Mild forms of autoimmune hepatitis may be more common than previously estimated. Low-level fluctuation of aminotransaminases, the presence of circulating autoantibodies, and mild histologic changes may only require observation, or low-dose pharmacologic monotherapy. More data are needed in this area.

A response to initial pharmacologic therapy is observed in 60% to 80% of cases, with a transplant-free survival at 10 years in excess of 90%. However, the survival advantage of medical therapy is more limited in patients with established cirrhosis (**Box 1**).

Pharmacologic Therapy

Of several agents with anti-inflammatory or immunosuppressive properties used for treatment of autoimmune hepatitis, corticosteroids and azathioprine have been the most extensively evaluated (see **Box 1**).[10–13] The indication to proceed with pharmacologic therapy is based primarily on the observation of an aggressive histologic picture on the liver biopsy, including interface hepatitis (also known as piecemeal or periportal necrosis). Patients with severe autoimmune hepatitis almost always have active interface hepatitis. Initial monotherapy with prednisone (or prednisolone) at doses of 40 to 60 mg/d in adults, is the preferred regime for patients with acute presentation of severe autoimmune hepatitis, when the prompt and potent anti-inflammatory effect of corticosteroids is needed.[14] In cases of moderate severity, lower doses of prednisone (15 to 30 mg/d), in combination with either azathioprine (50 to 150 mg/d) or 6-mercaptopurine (25 to 100 mg/d), can be employed as initial therapy. Whether monotherapy or in combination therapy, prednisone dose is gradually tapered over several weeks and months.

A common cause of relapse is an excessively rapid tapering of corticosteroids, leading to biochemical flare-ups or exacerbation.

The goal should be to achieve sustained biochemical remission (normalization of ALT) with the lowest possible dose of prednisone. Patients who achieve normal transaminases after a few weeks or months of therapy, should, in general, be maintained on therapy to complete at least 1 year of persistently normal ALT. A liver biopsy should

---

Box 1
Autoimmune and cholestatic liver diseases

Autoimmune hepatitis

Primary biliary cirrhosis

Primary sclerosing cholangitis

Overlap syndromes

then be repeated; persistence of histologic inflammation is an indication to continue immunosuppressive therapy for another 12 months or longer, depending on the extent of the residual inflammation. In patients who object to a repeat liver biopsy, the less established approach of discontinuing therapy and closely monitoring ALT levels for the first several years may be considered. Another approach is to discontinue prednisone after remission is achieved, and embark on maintenance monotherapy with azathioprine (or mycophenolic acid) for several years.

Although the histologic response may not correlate temporarily with the biochemical response, the evolution of serum aminotransaminases is a key marker for the clinician to assess response to therapy in autoimmune hepatitis. Other biochemical markers indicating improvement include a diminishing level of globulins and IgG, and in patients with hepatic synthetic dysfunction, the normalization of serum albumin, INR, and bilirubin. Titers of circulating autoantibodies, antinuclear antibodies, antismooth muscle antibodies are not generally useful to guide therapy in autoimmune hepatitis.

Once a patient has achieved remission for 1 to 2 years, the overall chance of maintaining remission after therapy is withdrawn is approximately 30% to 50%. Patients with established cirrhosis may require long-term therapy.

Some patients may have active and less responsive forms of the disease, characterized by decrease in ALT but lack of normalization despite robust doses of prednisone (≥ 20 mg/d), with or without azathioprine. Others have repeated relapses during tapering of corticosteroids, forcing increases to higher doses. In these patients, one may have to compromise and accept partial control of disease activity, generally defined as ALT at or less than 2 to 3 times the upper normal level, to avoid the severe side effects of long-term high-dose corticosteroids.

Lastly, a small but not insignificant group of patients fail to show any improvement after initial therapy with prednisone. The diagnosis needs to be re-evaluated but some of these patients may indeed have steroid-resistant forms of autoimmune hepatitis (see later discussion).

Patients with a mild form of autoimmune hepatitis, defined as modest elevation of ALT and inflammation without fibrosis, confined to the portal tracts on liver biopsy, can be observed while on no pharmacologic therapy initially. However, periodic monitoring of liver tests is mandatory as some patients may eventually develop florid autoimmune hepatitis and require therapy.

Certain therapeutic drugs have been reported to cause an autoimmune hepatitis, even when positive for antinuclear antibodies. For this reason, it seems prudent to advise patients with autoimmune hepatitis to avoid therapy with these drugs (examples include α-methyldopa, isoniazid, phenytoin, hydralazine, nitrofurantoin, minocycline).[15]

A suggested algorithm for the management of autoimmune hepatitis is presented in **Fig. 1**.

Autoimmune Hepatitis and Hepatitis C

A particularly troublesome situation occurs in patients with coexistent chronic hepatitis C virus infection and autoimmune hepatitis.[16–19] Prominent plasma cells on liver biopsy and high titer of autoantibodies in the setting of a positive serum hepatitis C RNA define this complex syndrome. No satisfactory management protocol has been validated or universally accepted for these individuals. In general, efforts should be made to determine if one of the diseases predominates. If features of autoimmune hepatitis are more prominent (abundant plasma cells, interface hepatitis, multiple autoantibodies at high titers, other associated autoimmune phenomena), a careful trial

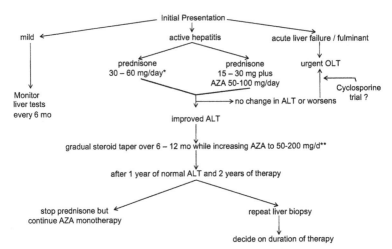

Fig. 1. Algorithm for the management of autoimmune hepatitis. Initial presentation is defined as *mild* if the patient is asymptomatic, with low-level elevation of transaminases, and inflammation is confined to the portal tracts on liver biopsy. *Active hepatitis* is defined as prominent interface hepatitis on biopsy, with or without serum ALT elevated to greater than 5 times the upper normal level in generally symptomatic patients. *Fulminant* presentation with acute liver failure is defined as the presence of hepatic encephalopathy and coagulopathy. AZA, azathioprine.*Prednisone at 30 mg/d for small persons or moderate disease severity; prednisone at 60 mg/d for large persons or severe disease activity. **Azathioprine monotherapy at 1.5–2.0 mg/kg/d, not to exceed 200 mg/d.

of anti-inflammatory and immunosuppressive therapy could be considered. In contrast, if hepatitis C virus infection is believed to be the dominant illness, our experience with interferon-based antiviral therapy has been generally negative, due to the risk of severe exacerbation of the autoimmune disease. In these circumstances, it might be better not to treat the viral disease. Nevertheless, this is a controversial and difficult area in hepatology; new approaches are clearly needed. Cyclosporin A, an immunosuppressive agent with some possible antiviral activity against hepatitis C, is a reasonable candidate for clinical trials of coexisting autoimmune hepatitis and hepatitis C virus infection.

Azathioprine

Azathioprine, a prodrug of mercaptopurine, is a key component of pharmacologic therapy for autoimmune hepatitis, as a steroid-sparing agent and in the maintenance phase of therapy. Azathioprine is not used as initial monotherapy to induce remission. Azathioprine is used as initial therapy as an adjunct to corticosteroids (prednisone or prednisolone). Doses can be gradually increased to 1 to 1.5 mg/kg/d provided the white cell count remains within an acceptable range. After corticosteroids are withdrawn, long-term monotherapy with azathioprine may maintain remission. Azathioprine is generally well tolerated but some patients may develop abdominal pain or other side effects limiting its tolerance.

Azathioprine and 6-mercaptopurine are methylated by thiopurine-methyl transferase, an enzyme associated with genetically determined heterogeneous levels of activity. However, the clinical value of thiopurine-methyl transferase genotype determination has not been established in the management of autoimmune hepatitis.

6-Mercaptopurine has been less studied than azathioprine in the management of autoimmune hepatitis.

Mycophenolate Mofetil

An increasing number of reports suggest that between 65% and 100% of patients intolerant or nonresponsive to prednisone with or without azathiprine, may achieve remission with mycophenolate mofetil (MMF).[20,21] Although promising, these series are mostly retrospective reviews of small numbers of patients. Nevertheless, the introduction of MMF in the management of autoimmune hepatitis represents a reasonable option for intolerant or nonresponsive patients. Reported dosages of MMF are 500 to 1,000 mg twice a day. MMF is generally well tolerated but adverse events may include vomiting, diarrhea, and leucopenia. A larger prospective evaluation of MMF is warranted to define its role in the management of autoimmune hepatitis.

Cyclosporine

Cyclosporine A, a calcineurin inhibitor, is widely used in post-transplant immunosuppression. As with mycophenolate, the role of cyclosporine, if any, remains undefined in autoimmune hepatitis.

On the basis of limited data, some clinicians perform a careful empirical trial of cyclosporine therapy in patients with severe, corticosteroid-resistant autoimmune hepatitis. The significant systemic toxicities of long-term cyclosporine therapy including renal toxicity should be kept in mind. Another potential role for cyclosporine is in patients with concurrent autoimmune hepatitis and chronic hepatitis C infection, given the modest antiviral activity of cyclosporine (see earlier discussion).

Other Agents

Reports of the use of tacrolimus, budesonide, methotrexate, ursodeoxycholic acid (UDCA), and cyclophosphamide are limited to case reports and small series of patients with autoimmune hepatitis.[13] The precise role of these agents in the management of autoimmune hepatitis is undefined. These pharmacologic agents could be cautiously considered in the occasional patient with severe, recalcitrant autoimmune hepatitis, who is also nonresponsive to or intolerant of prednisone, azathioprine, or MMF.

Liver Transplantation

Patients who develop decompensated cirrhosis despite immunosuppressive therapy can be successfully treated with liver transplantation.[14,22,23] Long-term survival after transplantation for autoimmune hepatitis is as good or better than transplantation for cirrhosis due to viral hepatitis. The clinical indications to begin a pretransplant evaluation are the same as for other liver diseases (refractory ascites, intractable hepatic encephalopathy, high Model for End-stage Liver Disease [MELD] score, hepatorenal syndrome, recurrent variceal hemorrhage). Hepatocellular carcinoma can complicate cirrhosis due to autoimmune hepatitis, even with good disease control by immunosuppressive therapy.

The variant of autoimmune hepatitis presenting with fulminant liver failure may not respond quickly or sufficiently to corticosteroids. Urgent liver transplantation may be necessary to prevent death due to acute liver failure.

Recurrence of autoimmune hepatitis after transplantation occurs in a minority of patients.[22–28] The diagnosis of recurrence can be difficult due to histopathologic features similar to chronic, relapsing, or acute allograft rejection. Some transplant centers use higher baseline immunosuppression in recipients transplanted for autoimmune hepatitis, hoping to minimize the risk of disease recurrence.

An autoimmunelike chronic hepatitis after transplantation for diseases other than autoimmune hepatitis has been reported sporadically.[25] This illness, better named alloimmune or allogeneic hepatitis, seems to respond well to corticosteroids and increased maintenance immunosuppression.

PRIMARY BILIARY CIRRHOSIS

Primary biliary cirrhosis (PBC) is a chronic and progressive cholestatic disease of the liver with a presumed autoimmune etiology. It is characterized by a T lymphocyte mediated attack on the small intrahepatic bile ducts, which results in progressive ductopenia. Cholestasis develops and advances slowly to fibrosis and cirrhosis. Although liver failure occurs gradually, patient survival is diminished compared with an age- and gender-matched population.[29,30]

PBC is diagnosed more frequently and at an earlier stage now than it was 10 years ago. It is not believed that this is due to a higher incidence of the disease, but rather that there is now greater recognition of the disease by physicians and more routine blood work, resulting in the detection of asymptomatic elevation of alkaline phosphatase and more widespread use of antimitochondrial antibody (AMA).[31] Most cases of PBC are diagnosed in asymptomatic patients who have been found to have hepatomegaly or an increased alkaline phosphatase level.[32] More than 95% of cases occur in women between the ages of 30 and 65. If symptomatic, fatigue and pruritus are the most common complaints.

AMA is detected in 95% of patients with PBC, and is the serologic hallmark of the disease. It has a specificity of 98% for PBC, and is arguably the most highly disease-specific autoantibody.[33] AMAs target 4 principal autoantigens, which have collectively been referred to as the M2 subtype of mitochondrial autoantigens: the E2 subunits of the pyruvate dehydrogenase complex, the branched chain 2-oxo-acid dehydrogenase complex, the ketoglutarate-dehydrogenase complex, and the hydrolipoamide dehydrogenase binding protein.[34] Each of these autoantigens participate in oxidative phosphorylation, a process by which ATP is formed. Most AMAs react against the E2 subunit of pyruvate dehydrogenase. A major advance in understanding the pathogenesis of PBC occurred with the identification and cloning of these antigens in 1988.[35] PBC is the only disease in which there are B and T cells that are autoreactive against the E2 subunit of pyruvate dehydrogenase. An AMA titer of 1:40 is usually enough to make the diagnosis of PBC; titers differ between patients, and do not correlate with disease severity or response to treatment. In addition to a positive AMA, serum IgM and total cholesterol may be elevated (**Box 2**).

A liver biopsy is not essential to make the diagnosis of PBC if the patient presents with typical symptoms and biochemical profile, and a positive AMA. A liver biopsy is usually performed to stage the disease and it may also show distinct histologic features highly suggestive of PBC, for example, portal mononuclear inflammation with granulomatous destruction of the bile ducts, and, if the disease is more advanced, fibrosis and cirrhosis (**Boxes 3 and 4**).

The treatment of PBC and its complications is discussed in detail later.

Treatment of Primary Biliary Cirrhosis

Unfortunately, there has been little success in treating the immunologic injury of the bile ducts in patients with PBC. Current treatment is limited to UDCA, the only approved therapy for PBC. The benefits of other therapies, such as methotrexate

---

Box 2
Pharmacologic agents for autoimmune hepatitis

Corticosteroids

Azathiprine

6-Mercaptopurine

Mycophenolate mofetil

Ursodiol

    Experimental

Budesonide

Cyclosporine

Tacrolimus

Rapamycin

Cyclophosphamide

Methotrexate

---

and colchicine, are unclear. Glucocorticoids and other immunosuppressive agents do not seem to improve the course of the disease.

Ursodeoxycholic acid

UDCA is a naturally occurring bile acid with choleretic properties. The initial trial by Poupon and colleagues[36] using 13–15 mg/kg/d of UDCA found significant decreases in alkaline phosphatase, bilirubin, ALT, and pruritus. This pioneer study led to several subsequent trials, including 5 large placebo-controlled trials[37–41] and 3 meta-analyses.[42–44]

In each of the placebo-controlled trials, patients received UDCA at a dose of 13 to 15 mg/kg/d and were followed for 2 to 6 years. The trials included between 145 and

---

Box 3
Abnormal serologic tests found in primary biliary cirrhosis

- Alanine aminotransferase (rarely greater than 5 times the upper limit of normal)
- Alkaline phosphatase (elevated)
- Antimitochondrial antibody (at titers greater than 1:40)
- Aspartate aminotransferase (rarely greater than 5 times the upper limit of normal)
- Bile acids (elevated)
- Cholesterol (total cholesterol may exceed 1,000 mg/dL. In early disease, high-density lipoprotein is elevated, low-density lipoprotein and very-low-density lipoprotein are mildly elevated. In cirrhosis, low-density lipoprotein is elevated and high-density lipoprotein is decreased)
- γ-Glutamyltransferase (elevated)
- IgM fraction of immunoglobulins (elevated)
- 5′-Nucleotidase (elevated)
- Total bilirubin (a poor prognostic sign)

> **Box 4**
> **Histologic stages of primary biliary cirrhosis**
>
> - Stage I—portal hepatitis with granulomatous destruction of the bile ducts
> - Stage II—periportal hepatitis and bile duct proliferation
> - Stage III—presence of fibrous septa or bridging necrosis
> - Stage IV—cirrhosis

222 patients. Only a few patients withdrew due to side effects. In all of the trials, there was a significant reduction in serum levels of alkaline phosphatase, bilirubin, aminotransferases, IgM, and cholesterol. The time to liver transplantation or death did not seem to be significantly improved after treatment with UDCA in the trials that only followed patients for 2 years, but when the patients were followed for 4 to 6 years, the probability of liver transplantation or death was significantly decreased. Histology improved in 2 trials[38,40] but in a larger analysis of 367 patients (200 who received UDCA and 167 on placebo) who had participated in 4 clinical trials, there was no significant difference in the histologic progression of disease except in the subgroup of patients that had early histologic stage at baseline (I or II).[45] This was consistent with another large, long-term trial by Combes and colleagues[37] in which only patients who presented with histologic stage I or II disease and a serum bilirubin level <2.0 mg/dL benefited from UDCA.

The meta-analyses yielded conflicting conclusions. In 2 of the meta-analyses, one of which included 16 randomized trials and the other 17 controlled trials, there was no effect on overall or transplant-free survival.[42,43] In the third meta-analysis, the investigators excluded studies of short duration (less than 2 years) and those that used doses of UDCA less than 10 mg/kg/d, and concluded that long-term UDCA significantly improved transplant-free survival and delayed histologic progression in early stage disease.[44] A decision analysis using a Markov model concluded that treatment with UDCA in the early stages of PBC (histologic stage I or II) was associated with survival similar to an age-matched control population (relative risk [RR], 0.8, $P = .5$) but the probability of death or liver transplantation was still increased in patients beginning treatment at later stages (RR, 2.2, $P \leq 0.05$).[46]

Given the data currently available and the safety profile of UDCA, it is recommended to treat patients with early stage PBC with UDCA at 13 to 15 mg/kg/d either in divided doses or a single daily dose. Biochemical markers of cholestasis are improved, pruritus may decrease, and the development of esophageal varices is delayed with UDCA therapy.[47] UDCA slows the progression of early PBC but does not cure it and patients ultimately still may progress to liver failure.

Azathioprine

Azathioprine is a purine synthesis inhibitor with immunosuppressive properties. It was studied in a large multicenter, double-blind, randomized trial that included 248 patients (127 received azathioprine and 121 received placebo).[48] This trial showed no benefit of treatment of PBC with azathioprine. These findings were supported by a recent Cochrane review which found that azathioprine did not significantly reduce mortality (RR, 0.80, 95% CI, 0.49–1.31) or improve pruritus (RR, 0.71, 95% CI, 0.28–1.84).[49] Given these data and the significant side effect profile of azathioprine, it is not recommended for use in PBC. Azathioprine may, however, be considered in the management of overlap syndrome between PBC and autoimmune hepatitis (see later discussion).

Prednisolone
Given the putative autoimmune nature of PBC, corticosteroids have been evaluated as therapy for PBC, but no clear benefit has been observed. A small placebo-controlled trial that followed 36 patients for 3 years reported decreased alkaline phosphatase levels but no change in overall mortality.[50] Steroids cannot be recommended for the treatment of PBC.

Cyclosporine
Cyclosporine is a calcineurin inhibitor and has been evaluated in 3 trials for the treatment of PBC.[51–53] The first 2 trials, which included only 12 and 19 patients followed for 1 year, reported a significant decrease in alkaline phosphatase but no improvement in histologic stage. There was a predictable increase in serum creatinine in both studies. These studies led to a larger multicenter placebo-controlled trial by Lombard and colleagues[51] in which 349 patients were randomized to receive cyclosporine at 3 mg/kg/d or placebo. Seventy-seven patients were followed for 6 years and, in a multivariate analysis, time to death or transplantation was significantly prolonged (by up to 50%) in the treatment arm of the study. Serum creatinine increased in the cyclosporine group in 9% of patients and the dose needed to be adjusted in 11% of patients. A Cochrane review concluded that there was no evidence that cyclosporine may delay death, time to liver transplantation, or progression of PBC, and given its significant side effect profile, was not recommended for use outside of clinical trials.[54]

Colchicine
Colchicine inhibits microtubule polymerization by binding to tubulin, ultimately preventing mitosis. Its mechanism of action in the treatment of PBC remains unknown, but it has been studied in several small studies with varying degrees of success.[55–58] Although there was improvement in serum biochemical parameters, there was no histologic improvement or survival benefit seen except in the trial by Kaplan and colleagues. A systematic review of 10 studies, which included 631 patients, also did not show any significant benefit on mortality, the need for liver transplantation, or improvement in biochemical tests or histology.[59]

A placebo-controlled trial of 90 patients compared colchicine with UDCA.[60] Pruritus was improved with both drugs. Colchicine improved liver biochemical tests slightly, whereas UDCA significantly reduced aminotransferases and alkaline phosphatase.

Methotrexate
Methotrexate inhibits the metabolism of folic acid and was first used in the treatment of PBC because of its encouraging effects on another cholestatic disease, primary sclerosing cholangitis. As with other PBC medications studied, there have been varying results in clinical trials with the use of methotrexate.[61–69] The largest multicenter controlled trial (the Primary Biliary Cirrhosis Ursodiol plus Methotrexate or its Placebo, or the PUMPS trial) found no benefit from the addition of methotrexate on transplant-free survival when patients were studied for a median period of 7.6 years.[70] A smaller study by Kaplan and colleagues[71] looked at the addition of methotrexate or colchicine to UDCA in 85 patients. There was no improvement in survival in any of the groups studied. Hence, there are insufficient data to support the use of methotrexate in the treatment of PBC.

Hepatocellular Carcinoma and Primary Biliary Cirrhosis

Previously, patients with PBC were considered to be at low risk for the development of hepatocellular carcinoma (HCC).[72] The frequency of HCC in PBC has been reported to be between 0.7% and 16%[73,74] It seems to occur more frequently in men than in women; in 1 study with 273 PBC patients with advanced disease, the overall incidence of HCC was 5.9%, the incidence was 4.1% in women, and 20% in men.[75] Older age (>70 years), male sex, history of blood transfusion, and signs of portal hypertension or cirrhosis are associated with HCC in patients with PBC.[76,77]

In a recent retrospective study at the Mayo Clinic, 36 patients with PBC were diagnosed with HCC between 1997 and 2007.[78] Seventeen of the patients were identified as part of a surveillance program and these patients were much more likely to undergo therapy and had an improved survival when compared with the patients diagnosed outside of the surveillance program. The investigators estimated the probability of development of HCC based on a predictive model that included older age (>70 years), male sex, history of blood transfusion, and any signs of portal hypertension or cirrhosis. Only 1 of the patients had less than a 6% probability of developing HCC. This study is important in that it not only shows the survival benefit of a surveillance program but also recommends that high risk patients should be screened for HCC. A noncirrhotic patient with PBC should not be part of a surveillance program for HCC.

Liver Transplantation for Primary Biliary Cirrhosis

The absolute number of transplants performed for PBC has decreased by an average of 5.4 cases per year ($P = .004$) and the number of patients listed for transplant for PBC has also decreased between 1995 and 2006.[79] This may reflect earlier diagnosis and institution of therapy for PBC.

The Mayo risk score is a mathematical model for predicting probability of survival in individual patients with PBC.[80] It uses the patient's age, total serum bilirubin and serum albumin concentrations, prothrombin time, and severity of edema. The formula for calculating the Mayo risk score is:

Risk = $0.971 \log_e$(bilirubin in mg/dL) + $2.53 \log_e$(albumin in g/dL) + 0.039 age in years + $2.38 \log_e$(prothrombin time in seconds) + $0.859 \log_e$(edema score of 0, 0.5, or 1.0) (http://www.mayoclinic.org/gi-rst/mayomodel2.html). However, the MELD predictive score, is used in practice to predict survival and the need for transplantation in patients with PBC.

Patients with PBC should be referred for transplant evaluation if 1 or more of the following are present: (1) The serum bilirubin level is greater than 5 mg/dL; (2) The serum albumin level is less than 2.8 g/dL; (3) Signs of portal hypertension (ascites, edema, variceal bleeding, encephalopathy); (4) MELD score approaching 15. In addition to the development of cirrhosis and liver failure from PBC, patients should also be considered for liver transplantation in cases of extreme debilitating pruritus or severe osteoporosis.

PBC may recur in the transplanted liver. A large cohort had recurrence in 16% of recipients at 5 years, and 30% at 10 years. A later report observed a recurrence rate of 23% at a median of 6.5 years.[81,82] However, despite recurrent disease, the rates of graft loss and the need for retransplantation are quite low.

Complications of Primary Biliary Cirrhosis

Patients with PBC progress at variable rates. Symptoms usually develop within 2 to 4 years in asymptomatic patients,[29] but up to one third of patients can remain asymptomatic for many years.[30] Pruritus can be a challenging common complaint, but patients also develop sicca syndrome, Raynaud syndrome, portal hypertension, metabolic bone disease, fat-soluble vitamin deficiency, and hypothyroidism.

Pruritus

Pruritus is the presenting symptom in approximately one third of patients diagnosed with PBC. Pruritus associated with PBC rarely disappears spontaneously and is worse at night, under constrictive clothing, with dry skin, and in hot and humid weather. At times the pruritus can be so severe as to cause sleep deprivation and affect quality of life sufficient enough to necessitate liver transplantation. The severity of the pruritus is not related to the severity of the PBC. The pathogenesis of this pruritus is unknown.

Treatment of pruritus from PBC can be extremely challenging. Topical therapies are ineffective and antihistamines are effective only at the early stages of the disease. The first choice of therapy is the anion-binding resin cholestyramine,[83] which has led to the theory that the pruritus is secondary to the sequestration of bile acids in the skin but this has not been confirmed.[84] Cholestyramine works best when taken before breakfast, and it is important to separate it from other medications by 2 to 4 hours as it will also bind oral medications. The initial dose of cholestyramine is 4 g three times a day and can be increased to a maximum of 16 g/d if needed. Pruritus usually remits within 2 to 4 days of starting therapy. Despite its benefits, many patients find taking cholestyramine unpleasant.

The use of UDCA for the treatment of pruritus is disappointing. In the trial by Heathcote and colleagues[38] in which 222 patients were treated with either UDCA at 14 mg/kg/d or placebo for 24 months, there was no improvement in pruritus. In 1 trial in which patients were treated with high-dose UDCA at 30 mg/kg/d there was improvement in pruritus.[85] A recent Cochrane analysis evaluated a combined total of 438 patients for improvement in pruritus while on UDCA without any beneficial effect seen (RR, 0.97, 95% CI, 0.78–1.19).[42]

Sertraline was recently studied in a small controlled trial by Mayo and colleagues[86] in which 12 patients received either sertraline or placebo. Patients on sertraline at doses between 75 and 100 mg had significant improvement in their pruritus scores ($P = .0009$). However, this study included any patient with cholestatic-associated pruritus and not just PBC patients. In a small retrospective study, 6/7 patients recorded an improvement in their pruritus severity while on sertraline; some patients were able to discontinue their anti-itching medication while on sertraline.[87]

Rifampin has shown promise for pruritus associated with cholestasis and should be considered as a third-line therapy.[88,89] The benefits of rifampin may be due to an alteration in the intracellular bile acid milieu. Side effects include an unconjugated hyperbilirubinemia, dark stained urine, and, uncommonly, hepatitis, thrombocytopenia, and renal tubular damage. The dose is 150 mg orally 2 to 3 times a day.

Opioid antagonists have been shown to be beneficial in the treatment of pruritus associated with chronic cholestasis. Nalmefene was first used with benefit, but narcotic withdrawal occurred in some patients[90]; this medication is not approved for this use. Naloxone is highly effective, but requires an intravenous route of administration and hence is not practical in clinical practice.[91] Naltrexone is an oral opioid antagonist that has been effective in clinical studies to ameliorate pruritus in up to 50% of patients, as well as symptoms of fatigue and depression.[92] Unfortunately it can lead to opioid-withdrawal symptoms and chronic pain (in patients who require opioids to treat pain syndromes).

Large volume plasmapheresis,[93] UDCA,[94] ultraviolet B light[95] and phenobarbital[96] have also been used with varying degrees of success. Unfortunately, often no treatment for pruritus is effective and patients require consideration for liver transplantation despite adequate synthetic function.

Sicca syndrome

Sicca syndrome is present in up to 86% of patients with PBC.[97,98] Sicca symptoms include dry eyes, dry mouth, dental caries, dysphagia, tracheobronchitis, and dyspareunia. It is most common in patients with CREST syndrome (calcinosis cutis, Raynaud disease, esophageal dysmotility, sclerodactyly, and telangiectasias), CREST syndrome in its complete form is rare in patients with PBC.[99]

It is important to directly question patients about sicca syndrome, as patients may not volunteer these symptoms. There is no cure for sicca syndrome, hence therapy is aimed at treating the symptoms. Artificial tears are used to treat the xerophthalmia. Patients should be counseled to visit the dentist regularly as a dry mouth can lead to an increase in dental caries. If dysphagia is present, all medications should be taken with plenty of water and in an upright position; other antireflux precautions should also be taken. Lubricating jelly or estrogen cream may be needed to treat dyspareunia in women post menopause.

Raynaud syndrome

Raynaud syndrome is a condition in which the fingers or the toes change color after exposure to temperature changes or emotional events. Pain can be particularly troublesome for patients living in colder climates. Smoking can increase the severity of the syndrome and patients should be advised to stop smoking. Calcium channel blockers are often prescribed to relieve symptoms.

Esophageal spasm

Painful esophageal spasms can occur in a minority of patients with PBC. The treatment involves treating any underlying acid reflux with antireflux medications and avoiding extremely hot or cold foods. If this is not successful, then smooth muscle relaxants, such as calcium-channel blockers or nitrates, or tricyclic antidepressants can be used.

Portal hypertension

Patients with PBC may present with variceal bleeding before the development of cirrhosis in contrast to most other liver diseases,[100,101] because of the early development of presinusoidal portal hypertension. If a patient is cirrhotic, then treatment of the portal hypertension should be as in any cirrhotic patient. If endoscopic (banding) therapy fails to control bleeding or recurrent hemorrhage, then transjugular intrahepatic portal systemic shunt (TIPS) is the next option. Splenorenal shunts were popular before the availability of TIPS but are dependent on local surgical expertise.[102]

Liver transplantation may be necessary in intractable symptomatic portal hypertension and is discussed in detail later.

Metabolic bone disease

Osteoporosis occurs 4 times more frequently in patients with PBC compared with age- and gender-matched controls.[103] Up to 30% of patients with PBC develop osteoporosis.[103,104] Decreased osteoblastic activity and increased osteoclastic activity contribute to the development of osteoporosis.[105] Patients may present with osteoporosis and be asymptomatic from their PBC; a patient with an elevated alkaline phosphatase and osteoporosis without fractures should be evaluated for the presence of PBC. In most cases, the development of osteoporosis is directly related to the duration and severity of PBC, and to the intensity and duration of jaundice. Metabolism of vitamin D is normal in PBC, but if there is malabsorption of calcium and vitamin D, this leads to osteoporosis. In addition, the presence of unconjugated hyperbilirubinemia has been found in in vitro models to prevent the proliferation and function of osteoblasts needed for bone formation.[106]

Treatment of osteoporosis includes bisphosphonate therapy and a daily dietary intake of 1,500 mg of calcium and 1,000 IU of vitamin D.[107–109] Neither treatment with UDCA nor calcitonin has been shown to benefit osteoporosis associated with PBC.[39,110] Vitamin D repletion alone has also not been shown to reduce the presence or severity of osteoporosis.[111] Severe osteoporosis may be an indication for liver transplantation, as improvement in bone density is seen as early as 6 months after transplantation.

Patients with PBC should undergo a baseline bone density scan at the time of diagnosis and then every 2 years thereafter. All patients should be advised to exercise regularly and stop smoking, as well as have an adequate intake of calcium and vitamin D. At the time of diagnosis, plasma concentrations of 25-hydroxyvitamin D, calcium, and phosphate should be obtained and repeated every 2 to 3 years. If vitamin D levels are normal, patients should take 800 IU/d of vitamin D; but, if the levels are low, vitamin D2 (ergocalciferol) should be tried at high doses, 50,000 IU orally 2 to 3 times/wk.[112] 25-Hydroxyvitamin D should be measured at 1 and 3 months while on these doses of vitamin D, and if levels normalize, patients should be switched to a maintenance dose of 800 IU/d.

If, after apparently adequate repletion with vitamin D, a patient remains vitamin D deficient, calcitriol can be used. Calcitriol is 1,25-dihydroxyvitamin D, a vitamin D metabolite. Calcitriol has a rapid onset of action and a half-life of only 6 hours. It is associated with a fairly high incidence of hypercalcemia and patients need to be followed closely while on therapy. Capsules are available in 20 and 50 μg doses. If using calcitriol as a supplement, 25-hydroxyvitamin D levels do not indicate clinical vitamin D status. Consultation with an endocrinologist with expertise in bone metabolism is advised for patients with significant osteopenia.

Fat-soluble vitamin deficiency
Patients with PBC who are jaundiced may have malabsorption of dietary fat, which may lead to steatorrhea, weight loss, and fat-soluble vitamin deficiencies. Steatorrhea reflects decreased biliary secretion of bile acids resulting in diminished concentrations of bile acids in the small intestine.[113] Treatment of steatorrhea includes a low-fat diet and, if needed, medium chain triglycerides, as their digestion and absorption of medium chain triglycerides are independent of the bile acid concentration. Most patients can tolerate 60 mL/d of medium chain triglycerides taken either by the teaspoon or used as salad dressing or a substitute for shortening in cooking.

Fat-soluble vitamins A, D, E, and K can be malabsorbed in PBC. Deficiency of vitamin K is often seen in severe cholestatic patients and the deficiency contributes to the coagulopathy caused by liver cell synthetic dysfunction. Thus, in advanced PBC, the prothrombin time is partially corrected by parenteral vitamin K (phytonadione), but vitamin E deficiency can occur in up to 13% of patients with PBC; it rarely has clinical significance in adults.[114] Vitamin A deficiency occurs in approximately 30% of patients, but is usually asymptomatic.[115] Vitamin A levels correlate directly with serum retinol binding protein and albumin levels, and indirectly with serum bilirubin levels. Vitamin A supplementation with 5,000 to 10,000 IU once or twice a week may be needed to correct vitamin A stores, but monitoring is important to prevent hypervitaminosis A and associated hepatotoxicity. Vitamin D deficiency should be addressed as described earlier. Annual measurement of vitamin A and 25-hydroxyvitamin D is recommended for patients with an elevated serum bilirubin;

measuring these levels every 2 to 3 years is sufficient in patients with normal serum bilirubin concentration.

Hypothyroidism

Approximately 20% of patients with PBC have, or will eventually develop, hypothyroidism.[116] The thyroid injury is believed to be autoimmune in nature. Treatment involves thyroid replacement therapy to maintain a normal serum thyroid stimulating hormone concentration.

PRIMARY SCLEROSING CHOLANGITIS

Primary sclerosing cholangitis (PSC) is a chronic, generally progressive, cholestatic liver disease characterized by obliterative fibrosis and inflammation of the large, medium, and small bile ducts. The cause of PSC remains obscure but genetic, autoimmune, and environmental factors are believed to participate in its pathogenesis. The diagnosis of PSC is based on cholangiographic features, after exclusion of secondary cholangiopathies. PSC is often associated with inflammatory bowel disease. Detailed reviews of the clinical features and natural history of PSC can be found elsewhere.[117–122]

The management of PSC often requires combined modalities, including pharmacologic agents, endoscopic procedures, and ultimately liver transplantation.[117]

Medical Management

The only drug extensively evaluated in PSC is UDCA.[123–125] It has been used in PSC based on its capacity to improve bile viscosity, thereby presumably decreasing bile plug formation and ameliorating secondary mechanisms of cholestatic cell damage.[126] However, early trials with standard doses of ursodiol (10–15 mg/kg/d) yielded modest, if any, improvement of biochemical abnormalities. Several reports using higher dosages of ursodiol (20–30 mg/kg/d) showed some improvement on the biochemical abnormalities of PSC.[124,125] However, a survival benefit could not be demonstrated. A large prospective trial with ursodiol at 17 to 23 mg/kg/d revealed a trend toward improved survival and decreased transplantation rate, but the outcome measures did not reach statistical significance.[125] Even though the study included 219 PSC patients, the sample size precluded reaching significance (or excluding a beneficial effect). A larger clinical trial of high-doses of ursodiol recently completed failed to show any clinical benefit in PSC, and has diminished the enthusiasm for this dose schedule in PSC.[126]

Endoscopic Management

The clinical course of PSC is unpredictable due to the highly variable segmental involvement. A patient may develop profound jaundice and cholestasis due to a single complete stricture strategically located at the junction of the intrahepatic biliary tree (a dominant stricture). Successful stenting and biliary dilatation may subsequently lead to rapid normalization of the biochemical tests and clinical features. Mechanical relief of biliary obstruction by endoscopic means can favorably affect prognosis and survival and have a key role in the management of PSC.[127] However, no comparative trials have been performed to identify a preferential endoscopic strategy in PSC. In general, the availability of sophisticated local endoscopic expertise is an important factor. The cholangiogram has to show discrete segmental stricture(s) in the extrahepatic or proximal right or left intrahepatic major ducts for endoscopic therapy to be feasible and potentially useful. Endoscopic therapy is not likely to help a PSC patient with a myriad of strictures diffusely affecting the central and peripheral smaller intrahepatic biliary branches. These patients would be better served by liver transplantation.

Due to strictures and bile stasis, biliary stones and sludge often form in PSC, which then contribute to biliary obstruction. Cholangioscopy can detect intraductal stones missed by cholangiography. Significant advances in biliary stent technology have reduced the need for nasobiliary drainage, with or without lavage with corticosteroids.

For patients with long, nonnegotiable strictures of extrahepatic ducts, transhepatic cholangiogram is the technique of choice to decompress and evaluate the biliary system. Percutaneous biliary tubes with periodic changes by interventional radiology have the potential to provide stabilization for prolonged periods of times. Key to endoscopic techniques in PSC is the ability to perform brushings, biopsies, and obtain cytologic material to screen and investigate cholangiocarcinoma. This malignancy can present in a manner indistinguishable from an otherwise benign PSC stricture. Cytologic biliary material should be obtained every time a patient with PSC undergoes endoscopic retrograde cholangiopancreatography.

Liver Transplantation for Primary Sclerosing Cholangitis

Disease-specific clinical indications for transplantation in PSC include the development of intractable severe pruritus, recurrent episodes of bacterial cholangitis or sepsis, and progressive severe bone disease. PSC patients can also develop end-stage complications similar to those observed in parenchymal liver failure, such as diuretic-resistant ascites, recurrent portal hypertensive bleeding, and intractable hepatic encephalopathy. In general, the MELD score is useful to assess prognosis and estimate survival in PSC. However, the MELD score may not adequately reflect disease severity in patients with cholestatic liver failure.

An unresolved issue is that of PSC patients who have dysplastic cells on biliary cytology obtained during periodic endoscopic retrograde cholangiopancreatography. There is concern that this represents possible transformation into cholangiocarcinoma. Once this malignancy is clinically apparent, transplantation is controversial because of a high rate of tumor recurrence post transplant. Effective methods for screening and early diagnosis of cholangiocarcinoma in PSC are urgently needed. Experimental protocols with preoperative external beam radiation and chemotherapy may expand the role of liver transplantation for cholangiocarcinoma.

OVERLAP SYNDROMES

Variants of autoimmune liver disease characterized by biochemical, serologic, and histologic features overlapping autoimmune hepatitis, PBC, and PSC are recognized.[128–132] Nomenclature for these syndromes is still evolving and has included terms such as antimitochondrial antibody-negative PBC, autoimmune cholangitis, autoimmune cholangiopathy, and others. The main overlap syndromes include autoimmune hepatitis overlapping with PBC, and autoimmune hepatitis associated with features of PSC. The clinical, biochemical, serologic and histopathologic features of overlap syndromes have been reviewed in detail elsewhere.[128–132]

Management

Due to the relative rarity of the overlap syndromes, no therapeutic, prospective, controlled clinical trials have been performed to establish optimal management. By extrapolation from therapies for autoimmune hepatitis, PBC, and PSC, clinicians often treat what seems to be the clinically dominant disease process in the overlap syndrome. Thus, if features of autoimmune hepatitis are more conspicuous than cholestasis, the initial approach may include anti-inflammatory and immunosuppressive agents.

Because of its benign safety profile and role in the management of PBC and PSC, ursodiol is often used as the initial therapy for the overlap syndrome. If significant clinical and biochemical responses are observed within a few months (resolution of pruritus or jaundice if present), bile acid therapy should be continued for the long term. As indicated earlier, if liver transaminases are substantially elevated, or interface hepatitis or fibrosis are prominent on the liver histology, initial management with corticosteroids plus azathioprine is appropriate, with ursodiol kept as a secondary agent. However, use of corticosteroids must be carefully justified and implemented with considerable caution in patients with overlap of autoimmune hepatitis and PSC due to the risks of bacterial cholangitis and sepsis.

Because of the lack of evidence-based data for guidance, management of patients with overlap syndromes is highly individualized and often based on empirical sequential use of combinations of immunosuppressants and ursodiol. The response of overlap syndromes to these therapies is quite variable, with some patients exhibiting satisfactory improvement, and others progressing to decompensated liver disease and requiring liver transplantation.

REFERENCES

1. Alvarez F, Berg PA, Bianchi FB, et al. International Autoimmune Hepatitis Group Report: review of criteria for diagnosis of autoimmune hepatitis. J Hepatol 1999; 31:929.
2. Krawitt EL. Autoimmune hepatitis. N Engl J Med 2006;354:54.
3. Krawitt EL. Clinical features and management of autoimmune hepatitis. World J Gastroenterol 2008;14:3301.
4. Lee WM, Seremba E. Etiologies of acute liver failure. Curr Opin Crit Care 2008; 14:198.
5. Kanzler S, Weidemann C, Gerken G, et al. Clinical significance of autoantibodies to soluble liver antigen in autoimmune hepatitis. J Hepatol 1999;31:635.
6. Czaja AJ. Understanding the pathogenesis of autoimmune hepatitis. Am J Gastroenterol 2001;96:1224.
7. Czaja AJ, Carpenter HA, Manns MP. Antibodies to soluble liver antigen, P450IID6, and mitochondrial complexes in chronic hepatitis. Gastroenterology 1993;105:1522.
8. Invernizzi P, Mackay IR. Autoimmune liver diseases. World J Gastroenterol 2008; 14:3290.
9. Choi G, Peters MG. The challenge of diagnosing autoimmune hepatitis: less is more. Hepatology 2008;48:10.
10. Luxon BA. Diagnosis and treatment of autoimmune hepatitis. Gastroenterol Clin North Am 2008;37:461.
11. Czaja AJ, Menon KV, Carpenter HA. Sustained remission after corticosteroid therapy for type 1 autoimmune hepatitis: a retrospective analysis. Hepatology 2002;35:890.
12. Mackay IR. Historical reflections on autoimmune hepatitis. World J Gastroenterol 2008;14:3292.
13. Soloway RD, Hewlett AT. The medical treatment for autoimmune hepatitis through corticosteroid to new immunosuppressive agents: a concise review. Ann Hepatol 2007;6:204.

14. Larsen FS. Treatment of patients with severe autoimmune hepatitis. Minerva Gastroenterol Dietol 2008;54:57.
15. Ford TJ, Dillon JF. Minocycline hepatitis. Eur J Gastroenterol Hepatol 2008;20: 796.
16. Bianchi FB, Muratori P, Granito A, et al. Hepatitis C and autoreactivity. Dig Liver Dis 2007;39(Suppl 1):S22.
17. Ferri C, Antonelli A, Mascia MT, et al. HCV-related autoimmune and neoplastic disorders: the HCV syndrome. Dig Liver Dis 2007;39(Suppl 1):S13.
18. Fried MW, Draguesku JO, Shindo M, et al. Clinical and serological differentiation of autoimmune and hepatitis C virus-related chronic hepatitis. Dig Dis Sci 1993; 38:631.
19. Strassburg CP, Vogel A, Manns MP. Autoimmunity and hepatitis C. Autoimmun Rev 2003;2:322.
20. Hennes EM, Oo YH, Schramm C, et al. Mycophenolate mofetil as second line therapy in autoimmune hepatitis? Am J Gastroenterol 2008;103:3063–70.
21. Inductivo-Yu I, Adams A, Gish RG, et al. Mycophenolate mofetil in autoimmune hepatitis patients not responsive or intolerant to standard immunosuppressive therapy. Clin Gastroenterol Hepatol 2007;5:799.
22. Ayata G, Gordon FD, Lewis WD, et al. Liver transplantation for autoimmune hepatitis: a long-term pathologic study. Hepatology 2000;32:185.
23. Narumi S, Hakamada K, Sasaki M, et al. Liver transplantation for autoimmune hepatitis: rejection and recurrence. Transplant Proc 1955;31:1999.
24. Gonzalez-Koch A, Czaja AJ, Carpenter HA, et al. Recurrent autoimmune hepatitis after orthotopic liver transplantation. Liver Transpl 2001;7:302.
25. Heffron TG, Smallwood GA, Oakley B, et al. Autoimmune hepatitis following liver transplantation: relationship to recurrent disease and steroid weaning. Transplant Proc 2002;34:3311.
26. Reich DJ, Fiel I, Guarrera JV, et al. Liver transplantation for autoimmune hepatitis. Hepatology 2000;32:693.
27. Salcedo M, Vaquero J, Banares R, et al. Response to steroids in de novo autoimmune hepatitis after liver transplantation. Hepatology 2002;35:349.
28. Tillmann HL, Jackel E, Manns MP. Liver transplantation in autoimmune liver disease—selection of patients. Hepatogastroenterology 1999;46:3053.
29. Balasubramaniam K, Grambsch PM, Wiesner RH, et al. Diminished survival in asymptomatic primary biliary cirrhosis. A prospective study. Gastroenterology 1990;98:1567.
30. Mahl TC, Shockcor W, Boyer JL. Primary biliary cirrhosis: survival of a large cohort of symptomatic and asymptomatic patients followed for 24 years. J Hepatol 1994;20:707.
31. Myszor M, James OF. The epidemiology of primary biliary cirrhosis in north-east England: an increasingly common disease? Q J Med 1990;75:377.
32. Prince MI, Chetwynd A, Craig WL, et al. Asymptomatic primary biliary cirrhosis: clinical features, prognosis, and symptom progression in a large population based cohort. Gut 2004;53:865.
33. Van de Water J, Cooper A, Surh CD, et al. Detection of autoantibodies to recombinant mitochondrial proteins in patients with primary biliary cirrhosis. N Engl J Med 1989;320:1377.
34. Kaplan MM, Gershwin ME. Primary biliary cirrhosis. N Engl J Med 2005;353:1261.
35. Coppel RL, McNeilage LJ, Surh CD, et al. Primary structure of the human M2 mitochondrial autoantigen of primary biliary cirrhosis: dihydrolipoamide acetyltransferase. Proc Natl Acad Sci U S A 1988;85:7317.

36. Poupon R, Chretien Y, Poupon RE, et al. Is ursodeoxycholic acid an effective treatment for primary biliary cirrhosis? Lancet 1987;1:834.

37. Combes B, Luketic VA, Peters MG, et al. Prolonged follow-up of patients in the U.S. multicenter trial of ursodeoxycholic acid for primary biliary cirrhosis. Am J Gastroenterol 2004;99:264.

38. Heathcote EJ, Cauch-Dudek K, Walker V, et al. The Canadian Multicenter Double-blind Randomized Controlled Trial of ursodeoxycholic acid in primary biliary cirrhosis. Hepatology 1994;19:1149.

39. Lindor KD, Dickson ER, Baldus WP, et al. Ursodeoxycholic acid in the treatment of primary biliary cirrhosis. Gastroenterology 1994;106:1284.

40. Pares A, Caballeria L, Rodes J, et al. Long-term effects of ursodeoxycholic acid in primary biliary cirrhosis: results of a double-blind controlled multicentric trial. UDCA-Cooperative Group from the Spanish Association for the Study of the Liver. J Hepatol 2000;32:561.

41. Poupon RE, Balkau B, Eschwege E, et al. A multicenter, controlled trial of urso-diol for the treatment of primary biliary cirrhosis. UDCA-PBC Study Group. N Engl J Med 1991;324:1548.

42. Gong Y, Huang Z, Christensen E, et al. Ursodeoxycholic acid for patients with primary biliary cirrhosis: an updated systematic review and meta-analysis of randomized clinical trials using Bayesian approach as sensitivity analyses. Am J Gastroenterol 2007;102:1799.

43. Goulis J, Leandro G, Burroughs AK. Randomised controlled trials of ursodeoxy-ycholic-acid therapy for primary biliary cirrhosis: a meta-analysis. Lancet 1999; 354:1053.

44. Shi J, Wu C, Lin Y, et al. Long-term effects of mid-dose ursodeoxycholic acid in primary biliary cirrhosis: a meta-analysis of randomized controlled trials. Am J Gastroenterol 2006;101:1529.

45. Poupon RE, Lindor KD, Pares A, et al. Combined analysis of the effect of treat-ment with ursodeoxycholic acid on histologic progression in primary biliary cirrhosis. J Hepatol 2003;39:12.

46. Corpechot C, Carrat F, Bahr A, et al. The effect of ursodeoxycholic acid therapy on the natural course of primary biliary cirrhosis. Gastroenterology 2005;128: 297.

47. Lindor KD, Jorgensen RA, Therneau TM, et al. Ursodeoxycholic acid delays the onset of esophageal varices in primary biliary cirrhosis. Mayo Clin Proc 1997;72: 1137.

48. Christensen E, Neuberger J, Crowe J, et al. Beneficial effect of azathioprine and prediction of prognosis in primary biliary cirrhosis. Final results of an interna-tional trial. Gastroenterology 1985;89:1084.

49. Gong Y, Christensen E, Gluud C. Azathioprine for primary biliary cirrhosis. Cochrane Database Syst Rev 2007;3:CD006000.

50. Mitchison HC, Palmer JM, Bassendine MF, et al. A controlled trial of predniso-lone treatment in primary biliary cirrhosis. Three-year results. J Hepatol 1992; 15:336.

51. Lombard M, Portmann B, Neuberger J, et al. Cyclosporin A treatment in primary biliary cirrhosis: results of a long-term placebo controlled trial. Gastroenterology 1993;104:519.

52. Minuk GY, Bohme CE, Burgess E, et al. Pilot study of cyclosporin A in patients with symptomatic primary biliary cirrhosis. Gastroenterology 1988;95:1356.

53. Wiesner RH, Ludwig J, Lindor KD, et al. A controlled trial of cyclosporine in the treatment of primary biliary cirrhosis. N Engl J Med 1990;322:1419.

54. Gong Y, Christensen E, Gluud C. Cyclosporin A for primary biliary cirrhosis. Cochrane Database Syst Rev 2007;3:CD005526.
55. Bodenheimer H Jr, Schaffner F, Pezzullo J. Evaluation of colchicine therapy in primary biliary cirrhosis. Gastroenterology 1988;95:124.
56. Kaplan MM, Alling DW, Zimmerman HJ, et al. A prospective trial of colchicine for primary biliary cirrhosis. N Engl J Med 1986;315:1448.
57. Warnes TW, Smith A, Lee FI, et al. A controlled trial of colchicine in primary biliary cirrhosis. Trial design and preliminary report. J Hepatol 1987;5:1.
58. Zifroni A, Schaffner F. Long-term follow-up of patients with primary biliary cirrhosis on colchicine therapy. Hepatology 1991;14:990.
59. Gong Y, Gluud C. Colchicine for primary biliary cirrhosis: a Cochrane Hepato-Biliary Group systematic review of randomized clinical trials. Am J Gastroenterol 2005;100:1876.
60. Vuoristo M, Farkkila M, Karvonen AL, et al. A placebo-controlled trial of primary biliary cirrhosis treatment with colchicine and ursodeoxycholic acid. Gastroenterology 1995;108:1470.
61. Babatin MA, Sanai FM, Swain MG. Methotrexate therapy for the symptomatic treatment of primary biliary cirrhosis patients, who are biochemical incomplete responders to ursodeoxycholic acid therapy. Aliment Pharmacol Ther 2006;24:813.
62. Bach N, Bodian C, Bodenheimer H, et al. Methotrexate therapy for primary biliary cirrhosis. Am J Gastroenterol 2003;98:187.
63. Bonis PA, Kaplan M. Methotrexate improves biochemical tests in patients with primary biliary cirrhosis who respond incompletely to ursodiol. Gastroenterology 1999;117:395.
64. Buscher HP, Zietzschmann Y, Gerok W. Positive responses to methotrexate and ursodeoxycholic acid in patients with primary biliary cirrhosis responding insufficiently to ursodeoxycholic acid alone. J Hepatol 1993;18:9.
65. Hendrickse MT, Rigney E, Giaffer MH, et al. Low-dose methotrexate is ineffective in primary biliary cirrhosis: long-term results of a placebo-controlled trial. Gastroenterology 1999;117:400.
66. Kaplan MM, DeLellis RA, Wolfe HJ. Sustained biochemical and histologic remission of primary biliary cirrhosis in response to medical treatment. Ann Intern Med 1997;126:682.
67. Kaplan MM, Knox TA. Treatment of primary biliary cirrhosis with low-dose weekly methotrexate. Gastroenterology 1991;101:1332.
68. Kaplan MM, Schmid C, Provenzale D, et al. A prospective trial of colchicine and methotrexate in the treatment of primary biliary cirrhosis. Gastroenterology 1999;117:1173.
69. Lindor KD, Dickson ER, Jorgensen RA, et al. The combination of ursodeoxycholic acid and methotrexate for patients with primary biliary cirrhosis: the results of a pilot study. Hepatology 1995;22:1158.
70. Combes B, Emerson SS, Flye NL, et al. Methotrexate (MTX) plus ursodeoxycholic acid (UDCA) in the treatment of primary biliary cirrhosis. Hepatology 2005;42:1184.
71. Kaplan MM, Cheng S, Price LL, et al. A randomized controlled trial of colchicine plus ursodiol versus methotrexate plus ursodiol in primary biliary cirrhosis: ten-year results. Hepatology 2004;39:915.
72. Johnson PJ, Krasner N, Portmann B, et al. Hepatocellular carcinoma in Great Britain: influence of age, sex, HBsAg status, and aetiology of underlying cirrhosis. Gut 1978;19:1022.

73. Deutsch M, Papatheodoridis GV, Tzakou A, et al. Risk of hepatocellular carcinoma and extrahepatic malignancies in primary biliary cirrhosis. Eur J Gastroenterol Hepatol 2008;20:5.

74. Turissini SB, Kaplan MM. Hepatocellular carcinoma in primary biliary cirrhosis. Am J Gastroenterol 1997;92:676.

75. Jones DE, Metcalf JV, Collier JD, et al. Hepatocellular carcinoma in primary biliary cirrhosis and its impact on outcomes. Hepatology 1997;26:1138.

76. Shibuya A, Tanaka K, Miyakawa H, et al. Hepatocellular carcinoma and survival in patients with primary biliary cirrhosis. Hepatology 2002;35:1172.

77. Suzuki A, Lymp J, Donlinger J, et al. Clinical predictors for hepatocellular carcinoma in patients with primary biliary cirrhosis. Clin Gastroenterol Hepatol 2007;5:259.

78. Silveira MG, Suzuki A, Lindor KD. Surveillance for hepatocellular carcinoma in patients with primary biliary cirrhosis. Hepatology 2008;48:1149.

79. Lee J, Belanger A, Doucette JT, et al. Transplantation trends in primary biliary cirrhosis. Clin Gastroenterol Hepatol 2007;5:1313.

80. Dickson ER, Grambsch PM, Fleming TR, et al. Prognosis in primary biliary cirrhosis: model for decision making. Hepatology 1989;10:1.

81. Liermann Garcia RF, Evangelista Garcia C, McMaster P, et al. Transplantation for primary biliary cirrhosis: retrospective analysis of 400 patients in a single center. Hepatology 2001;33:22.

82. Neuberger J, Gunson B, Hubscher S, et al. Immunosuppression affects the rate of recurrent primary biliary cirrhosis after liver transplantation. Liver Transpl 2004;10:488.

83. Datta DV, Sherlock S. Treatment of pruritus of obstructive jaundice with cholestyramine. Br Med J 1963;1:216.

84. Ghent CN, Bloomer JR, Klatskin G. Elevations in skin tissue levels of bile acids in human cholestasis: relation to serum levels and to pruritus. Gastroenterology 1977;73:1125.

85. Matsuzaki Y, Tanaka N, Osuga T, et al. Improvement of biliary enzyme levels and itching as a result of long-term administration of ursodeoxycholic acid in primary biliary cirrhosis. Am J Gastroenterol 1990;85:15.

86. Mayo MJ, Handem I, Saldana S, et al. Sertraline as a first-line treatment for cholestatic pruritus. Hepatology 2007;45:666.

87. Browning J, Combes B, Mayo MJ. Long-term efficacy of sertraline as a treatment for cholestatic pruritus in patients with primary biliary cirrhosis. Am J Gastroenterol 2003;98:2736.

88. Bachs L, Pares A, Elena M, et al. Effects of long-term rifampicin administration in primary biliary cirrhosis. Gastroenterology 1992;102:2077.

89. Ghent CN, Carruthers SG. Treatment of pruritus in primary biliary cirrhosis with rifampin. Results of a double-blind, crossover, randomized trial. Gastroenterology 1988;94:488.

90. Thornton JR, Losowsky MS. Opioid peptides and primary biliary cirrhosis. BMJ 1988;297:1501.

91. Bergasa NV, Alling DW, Talbot TL, et al. Effects of naloxone infusions in patients with the pruritus of cholestasis. A double-blind, randomized, controlled trial. Ann Intern Med 1995;123:161.

92. Wolfhagen FH, Sternieri E, Hop WC, et al. Oral naltrexone treatment for cholestatic pruritus: a double-blind, placebo-controlled study. Gastroenterology 1997;113:1264.

93. Cohen LB, Ambinder EP, Wolke AM, et al. Role of plasmapheresis in primary biliary cirrhosis. Gut 1985;26:291.

94. Poupon RE, Poupon R, Balkau B. Ursodiol for the long-term treatment of primary biliary cirrhosis. The UDCA-PBC Study Group. N Engl J Med 1994;330:1342.
95. Cerio R, Murphy GM, Sladen GE, et al. A combination of phototherapy and cholestyramine for the relief of pruritus in primary biliary cirrhosis. Br J Dermatol 1987;116:265.
96. Becker M, von Bergmann K, Rotthauwe HW, et al. Effects of phenobarbital on biliary lipid metabolism in children with chronic intrahepatic cholestasis. Eur J Pediatr 1984;143:41.
97. Giovannini A, Ballardini G, Amatetti S, et al. Patterns of lacrimal dysfunction in primary biliary cirrhosis. Br J Ophthalmol 1985;69:832.
98. Mang FW, Michieletti P, O'Rourke K, et al. Primary biliary cirrhosis, sicca complex, and dysphagia. Dysphagia 1997;12:167.
99. Reynolds TB, Denison EK, Frankl HD, et al. Primary biliary cirrhosis with scleroderma, Raynaud's phenomenon and telangiectasia. New syndrome. Am J Med 1971;50:302.
100. Navasa M, Pares A, Bruguera M, et al. Portal hypertension in primary biliary cirrhosis. Relationship with histological features. J Hepatol 1987;5:292.
101. Thornton JR, Triger DR, Losowsky MS. Variceal bleeding is associated with reduced risk of severe cholestasis in primary biliary cirrhosis. Q J Med 1989;71:467.
102. Boyer TD, Kokenes DD, Hertzler G, et al. Effect of distal splenorenal shunt on survival of patients with primary biliary cirrhosis. Hepatology 1994;20:1482.
103. Springer JE, Cole DE, Rubin LA, et al. Vitamin D-receptor genotypes as independent genetic predictors of decreased bone mineral density in primary biliary cirrhosis. Gastroenterology 2000;118:145.
104. Menon KV, Angulo P, Weston S, et al. Bone disease in primary biliary cirrhosis: independent indicators and rate of progression. J Hepatol 2001;35:316.
105. Hodgson SF, Dickson ER, Wahner HW, et al. Bone loss and reduced osteoblast function in primary biliary cirrhosis. Ann Intern Med 1985;103:855.
106. Janes CH, Dickson ER, Okazaki R, et al. Role of hyperbilirubinemia in the impairment of osteoblast proliferation associated with cholestatic jaundice. J Clin Invest 1995;95:2581.
107. Guanabens N, Pares A, Ros I, et al. Alendronate is more effective than etidronate for increasing bone mass in osteopenic patients with primary biliary cirrhosis. Am J Gastroenterol 2003;98:2268.
108. Wolfhagen FH, van Buuren HR, den Ouden JW, et al. Cyclical etidronate in the prevention of bone loss in corticosteroid-treated primary biliary cirrhosis. A prospective, controlled pilot study. J Hepatol 1997;26:325.
109. Zein CO, Jorgensen RA, Clarke B, et al. Alendronate improves bone mineral density in primary biliary cirrhosis: a randomized placebo-controlled trial. Hepatology 2005;42:762.
110. Camisasca M, Crosignani A, Battezzati PM, et al. Parenteral calcitonin for metabolic bone disease associated with primary biliary cirrhosis. Hepatology 1994;20:633.
111. Matloff DS, Kaplan MM, Neer RM, et al. Osteoporosis in primary biliary cirrhosis: effects of 25-hydroxyvitamin D3 treatment. Gastroenterology 1982;83:97.
112. Dawson-Hughes B, Heaney RP, Holick MF, et al. Estimates of optimal vitamin D status. Osteoporos Int 2005;16:713.
113. Lanspa SJ, Chan AT, Bell JS 3rd, et al. Pathogenesis of steatorrhea in primary biliary cirrhosis. Hepatology 1985;5:837.
114. Munoz SJ, Heubi JE, Balistreri WF, et al. Vitamin E deficiency in primary biliary cirrhosis: gastrointestinal malabsorption, frequency and relationship to other lipid-soluble vitamins. Hepatology 1989;9:525.

115. Phillips JR, Angulo P, Petterson T, et al. Fat-soluble vitamin levels in patients with primary biliary cirrhosis. Am J Gastroenterol 2001;96:2745.
116. Elta GH, Sepersky RA, Goldberg MJ, et al. Increased incidence of hypothyroidism in primary biliary cirrhosis. Dig Dis Sci 1983;28:971.
117. Charatcharoenwitthaya P, Lindor KD. Primary sclerosing cholangitis: diagnosis and management. Curr Gastroenterol Rep 2006;8:75.
118. Cullen SN, Chapman RW. Review article: current management of primary sclerosing cholangitis. Aliment Pharmacol Ther 2005;21:933.
119. Mendes FD, Lindor KD. Primary sclerosing cholangitis. Clin Liver Dis 2004;8: 195.
120. Silveira MG, Lindor KD. Primary sclerosing cholangitis. Can J Gastroenterol 2008;22:689.
121. Tischendorf JJ, Geier A, Trautwein C. Current diagnosis and management of primary sclerosing cholangitis. Liver Transpl 2008;14:735.
122. Weismuller TJ, Wedemeyer J, Kubicka S, et al. The challenges in primary sclerosing cholangitis–aetiopathogenesis, autoimmunity, management and malignancy. J Hepatol 2008;48(Suppl 1):S38.
123. Harnois DM, Angulo P, Jorgensen RA, et al. High-dose ursodeoxycholic acid as a therapy for patients with primary sclerosing cholangitis. Am J Gastroenterol 2001;96:1558.
124. Mitchell SA, Bansi DS, Hunt N, et al. A preliminary trial of high-dose ursodeoxycholic acid in primary sclerosing cholangitis. Gastroenterology 2001;121:900.
125. Olsson R, Boberg KM, de Muckadell OS, et al. High-dose ursodeoxycholic acid in primary sclerosing cholangitis: a 5-year multicenter, randomized, controlled study. Gastroenterology 2005;129:1464.
126. Lindor K, Enders F, Schmoll J, et al. Randomized, double-blind, controlled trial of high-dose ursodeoxycholic acid (UDCA) for primary sclerosing cholangitis. Hepatology 2008;48(Suppl 4):378A.
127. Baluyut AR, Sherman S, Lehman GA, et al. Impact of endoscopic therapy on the survival of patients with primary sclerosing cholangitis. Gastrointest Endosc 2001;53:308.
128. Mishima S, Omagari K, Ohba K, et al. Clinical implications of antimitochondrial antibodies in type 1 autoimmune hepatitis: a longitudinal study. Hepatogastroenterology 2008;55:221.
129. Premoli A, Morello E, Bo S, et al. Diagnostic and therapeutic questions in overlap syndromes of autoimmune hepatitis. Minerva Gastroenterol Dietol 2007;53: 79.
130. Rust C, Beuers U. Overlap syndromes among autoimmune liver diseases. World J Gastroenterol 2008;14:3368.
131. Sherlock S. Primary biliary cirrhosis, primary sclerosing cholangitis, and autoimmune cholangitis. Clin Liver Dis 2000;4:97.
132. van Buuren HR, van Hoogstraten HJE, Terkivatan T, et al. High prevalence of autoimmune hepatitis among patients with primary sclerosing cholangitis. J Hepatol 2000;33:543.

Hepatitis Vaccination and Prophylaxis

Carolyn T. Nguyen, BSN, MSN, CRNP[a], Tram T. Tran, MD[b],*

KEYWORDS

- Hepatitis A • Hepatitis B • Hepatitis C • Vaccinations
- Prophylaxis • Viral hepatitis

The 3 most commonly identified causes of viral hepatitis in the United States are hepatitis A virus (HAV), hepatitis B virus (HBV), and hepatitis C virus (HCV). Worldwide, approximately 1.4 million cases of acute HAV occur annually. Two billion people have been infected with HBV, and more than 350 million have chronic infection, with 600,000 dying each year from HBV-related liver disease or hepatocellular carcinoma. An estimated 130 million people have chronic hepatitis C worldwide. Each of these unrelated viruses can produce an acute illness characterized by nausea, malaise, abdominal pain, and jaundice. Acute infection with acute HBV and HCV can also lead to chronic infection, with an increased risk for cirrhosis and hepatocellular carcinoma. Safe and effective vaccines have been available for hepatitis B since 1981 and for hepatitis A since 1995. No vaccine is currently licensed against hepatitis C.[1]

HEPATITIS A

Hepatitis A is a self-limited disease that can result in fulminant hepatitis with acute liver failure, although death occurs in less than 1% of infected individuals.[2] The World Health Organization estimates an annual total of 1.5 million clinical cases of hepatitis A worldwide (**Box 1**).[3] Currently in the United States, there are only approximately 100 reported deaths annually from acute hepatitis A infection, with about 50% of the fatalities occurring in patients with pre-existing chronic liver disease.[4] However, it remains a significant cause of morbidity and socioeconomic loss in many parts of the world. HAV is transmitted from person to person via the fecal-oral route, as it is abundantly excreted in feces and can survive in the environment for prolonged periods of time; it is typically acquired by ingestion of contaminated food or water. Occasionally, HAV is also acquired through sexual contact (anal-oral) and blood transfusion. In areas where

a Division of Gastroenterology, Department of Medicine, Cedars-Sinai Medical Center, 8635 W. 3rd Street, Suite 1060W, Los Angeles, CA 90048, USA
b Department of Medicine, Geffen UCLA School of Medicine, Cedars-Sinai Medical Center, 8635 W. 3rd Street, Suite 590W, Los Angeles, CA 90048, USA
* Corresponding author.
E-mail address: trant@cshs.org (T.T. Tran).

Clin Liver Dis 13 (2009) 317–329
doi:10.1016/j.cld.2009.02.005
1089-3261/09/$ – see front matter © 2009 Elsevier Inc. All rights reserved.

liver.theclinics.com

Box 1
Groups at high risk for contracting hepatitis A

- People in household/sexual contact with infected persons
- Medical and paramedical personnel in hospitals
- International travelers from developed countries to regions of the world where HAV is endemic
- Persons living in regions with endemic hepatitis A
- Persons residing in areas where extended community outbreaks exist
- Preschool children attending day care centers, their parents, and siblings
- Day care center employees
- Residents and staff of closed communities (institutions)
- Men who have sex with men
- Drug users using unsterilized injection needles

HAV is highly endemic, most HAV infections occur during early childhood. With improved sanitation and hygiene, infection and natural immunity do not occur in childhood, and consequently, the number of adults susceptible to the disease increases. Under these conditions, explosive epidemics can arise from fecal contamination of a single source.[5]

Groups at Increased Risk for Hepatitis A

Travelers
Persons from the developed world who travel to developing countries are at substantial risk for acquiring hepatitis A. These people include tourists, immigrants and their children returning to their country of origin to visit friends or relatives, military personnel, missionaries, and others who work or study abroad in countries that have high or intermediate endemicity of hepatitis A. Hepatitis A remains one of the most common vaccine-preventable diseases acquired during travel. In the United States, children account for approximately 50% of reported travel-related cases. Travelers who acquire hepatitis A during their trips may also transmit HAV to contacts on their return.

Men who have sex with men
Cyclic outbreaks among men who have sex with men (MSM) have occurred in urban areas in the United States, Canada, Europe, and Australia. Since 1996, the Advisory Committee on Immunization Practices (ACIP) has recommended hepatitis A vaccination of MSM.

Users of injection and noninjection drugs
During the preceding 2 decades, outbreaks have been reported with increasing frequency among users of injection and noninjection drugs in Australia, Europe, and North America. Transmission among injection-drug users probably occurs through both percutaneous and fecal-oral routes. Since 1996, ACIP has recommended hepatitis A vaccination of users of illicit drugs.

Persons with clotting-factor disorders
During 1992 to 1993, outbreaks of hepatitis A were reported in Europe among persons with clotting-factor disorders who had been administered solvent-detergent-treated,

factor VIII concentrates that presumably had been contaminated from plasma donors incubating hepatitis A. Changes in viral inactivation procedures, high hepatitis A vaccine coverage, and improved donor screening have decreased the risk for HAV transmission from clotting factors.

Persons working with nonhuman primates
Outbreaks of hepatitis A have been reported among persons working with nonhuman primates that are susceptible to HAV infection. Primates that were infected were those that had been born in the wild, not those born and raised in captivity.

Food-service establishments and food handlers
Outbreaks are typically associated with contamination of food during preparation by an HAV-infected food handler; a single infected food handler can transmit HAV to dozens or even hundreds of persons. However, the majority of food handlers with hepatitis A do not transmit HAV. Food handlers are not at increased risk for hepatitis A because of their occupation. Outbreaks associated with food, especially green onions and other raw produce, that has been contaminated before reaching a food-service establishment have been recognized.

Child care centers
Outbreaks among children attending child care centers and persons employed at these centers have been recognized since the 1970s, but their frequency has decreased as overall hepatitis A incidence among children has declined in recent years. Because infection among children is typically mild or asymptomatic, outbreaks are often identified only when adult contacts (typically parents) become ill. Poor hygiene among children who wear diapers and the handling and changing of diapers by staff contribute to spread of HAV infection. Disease in child care centers more commonly reflects extended transmission from the community.

Health care institutions
Outbreaks of hepatitis A caused by transmission from adult patients to health-care workers are typically associated with fecal incontinence. Occasional outbreaks have occurred in neonatal intensive-care units because of infants acquiring infection from transfused blood and subsequently transmitting hepatitis A to other infants and staff.

Institutions for persons with developmental disabilities
Previously HAV infection was highly endemic in institutions for persons with developmental disabilities. As fewer children are institutionalized and as conditions in institutions have improved, the incidence and prevalence of HAV infection have decreased, although outbreaks still occur in these settings.

Hepatitis A in persons with chronic liver disease
Although not at increased risk for HAV infection, persons with chronic liver disease are at increased risk for fulminant hepatitis with hepatitis A superinfection, which can lead to overt hepatic decompensation.[5] Patients with acute hepatitis A superimposed on chronic hepatitis B infection have a more severe clinical course and higher death rate compared with that of otherwise healthy individuals with hepatitis A monoinfection, as reported in a large outbreak of acute hepatitis A in Shanghai in the late 1980s.[6] Similarly, patients with acute hepatitis A superinfection and chronic hepatitis C have increased risk of fatal fulminant hepatitis.[7] Recognition of chronic liver disease is an indication for vaccination against HAV.

Schools

In the United States, the occurrence of cases of hepatitis A in elementary or secondary schools typically reflects the prevalence of hepatitis A in the community.

Advisory Committee on Immunization Practices Recommendations

In 1996, the Centers for Disease Control and Prevention's (CDC) ACIP recommended administration of hepatitis A vaccine to persons at increased risk of infection, including international travelers, MSM, injection- and noninjection-drug users, and children living in communities with high rates of disease.[8] In 2006, the ACIP recommended hepatitis A vaccination of all children at age 12 to 23 months and catch-up vaccination of persons at increased risk for hepatitis A (eg, travelers to endemic areas, users of illicit drugs, or MSM).[8]

In June 2007, the ACIP included updated recommendations for prevention of hepatitis A after exposure to HAV. For decades, immunoglobulin (IG) has been recommended for prophylaxis after exposure to HAV.[9] IG is a sterile preparation of concentrated antibodies (IGs) made from pooled human plasma processed by cold ethanol fractionation. IG provides protection against hepatitis A through passive transfer of antibody. No transmission of HBV, human immunodeficiency virus (HIV), HCV, or other viruses has been reported from administration of intramuscular (IM) IG. When administered for pre-exposure prophylaxis, 1 dose of 0.02 mL/kg IM confers protection for less than 3 months, and 1 dose of 0.06 mL/kg IM confers protection for 3 to 5 months. When administered within 2 weeks after an exposure to HAV (0.02 mL/kg IM), IG is 80% to 90% effective in preventing hepatitis A. Efficacy is greatest when IG is administered early in the incubation period; when administered later in the incubation period, IG might only attenuate the clinical expression of HAV infection.[9]

For postexposure prophylaxis, persons who have recently been exposed to HAV and who previously have not received hepatitis A vaccine should be administered a single dose of single-antigen hepatitis A vaccine or IG (0.02 mL/kg) as soon as possible. For healthy persons aged 12 months to 40 years, single-antigen hepatitis A vaccine at the age-appropriate dose is preferred. For persons older than 40 years, IG is preferred; vaccine can be used if IG cannot be obtained. For children younger than 12 months, immunocompromised persons, persons who have had chronic liver disease diagnosed, and persons for whom vaccine is contraindicated, IG should be used.[9]

All susceptible persons traveling or working in countries that have high or intermediate hepatitis A endemicity should be vaccinated or receive IG before departure. Hepatitis A vaccine at age-appropriate dose is preferred to IG and should be administered as soon as travel is considered. One dose of single-antigen hepatitis A vaccine administered at any time before departure can provide adequate protection for most healthy persons. Older adults, immunocompromised persons, and persons with chronic liver disease or other chronic medical conditions planning to depart to an area in 2 weeks or less than 2 weeks should receive the initial dose of vaccine and also simultaneously can be administered IG (0.02 mL/kg) at a separate injection site. Travelers who elect not to receive vaccine, are aged younger than 12 months, or are allergic to a vaccine component should receive a single dose of IG (0.02 mL/kg), which provides effective protection for up to 3 months.[9]

Hepatitis A Vaccine

All children should receive hepatitis A vaccine at 1 year (ie, 12–23 months), with the first dose at the 12- to 15-month visit and the second dose, 6 to 12 months later. Children not vaccinated by 2 years of age can be vaccinated at later visits. Existing programs to immunize high-risk groups, such as MSM, injection-drug users, persons with liver disease, and those with clotting disorders, will continue. The hepatitis A vaccine is available as a single-antigen vaccine (Vaqta, Havrix) for children 12 months and older and in combination with hepatitis B vaccine (Twinrix) for those older than 18 years.[10]

HEPATITIS B

HBV can be transmitted vertically, through sexual or household contact, or by unsafe injections, but chronic infections acquired during infancy or childhood account for a disproportionately large number of worldwide morbidity and mortality. The prevalence of HBV infection is uneven throughout the world, with large burdens in Asia and the Pacific Islands, sub-Saharan Africa, the Amazon Basin, and Eastern Europe.[11] Vaccination against HBV infection can be started at birth, and it provides long-term protection against infection in more than 90% of healthy people.[12] After immunization, a serum titer of antibodies to hepatitis B surface antigen (HBsAg) (anti-HBs) of greater than or equal to 10 mIU/mL has been shown to be effective in preventing infection and is the generally accepted level for determining that a vaccine response has occurred.[13]

Hepatitis B vaccination is highly effective in preventing infection with HBV and consequent acute and chronic liver disease. First licensed in the United States in 1981, hepatitis B vaccine is now one of the most widely used vaccines in the world. It was also the world's first cancer prevention vaccine and the first vaccine to prevent a sexually transmitted disease (STD).[12] In the United States, the number of newly acquired HBV infections has declined substantially as a result of the implementation of a comprehensive national immunization program. However, the prevalence of chronic HBV infection remains high. In 2006, approximately 800,000 to 1.4 million US residents were living with chronic HBV infection, and hepatitis B is the underlying cause of an estimated 2,000 to 4,000 deaths each year in the United States.[14] Approximately 0.3% to 0.5% of US residents are chronically infected with HBV; 47% to 70% of these persons were born in other countries.[14] These immigrants are also from areas of high and intermediate endemicity. Approximately, 60% of the world's population lives in areas where HBV infection is highly endemic, including Asia and Africa. Southern Europe, the Middle East, and South Asia have an intermediate level of HBV endemicity.[12] The most effective way to prevent transmission of HBV is by immunization.

Indications

The national strategy to eliminate HBV transmission in the United States includes universal vaccination of infants beginning at birth (**Box 2**). Prevention of perinatal HBV infection requires routine screening of all pregnant women for HBsAg and immunoprophylaxis of infants born to HBsAg-positive women and infants born to women with unknown HBsAg status. Vaccination strategies also attempt to identify adults at increased risk of infection.[15] These adults include those with household contact and those who are intimate partners of HBV-infected persons; persons born in countries with HBsAg prevalence greater than or equal to 8%; postexposure prophylaxis (eg, needlestick injury to a health-care worker or sexual assault); and persons infected with HIV.[1] The CDC also recently issued major updates to the recommendations and approaches to address challenges in implementing the strategy to eliminate HBV transmission in the United States. These include the following measures: (1) improve prevention of perinatal and early childhood HBV transmission; (2) broaden vaccine coverage of children and adolescents not previously vaccinated; (3) provide universal

---

Box 2
Indications for pre-exposure hepatitis B vaccination

Universal

- All infants
- All children and adolescents not previously vaccinated

On the Basis of Risk

- Inmates of long-term correctional facilities
- Injection-drug users
- Sexually active MSM
- Men and women with more than 1 partner in the previous 6 months, a history of STD, or treatment in an STD clinic
- Household contacts (including cell mates) and sex partners of persons with chronic HBV infection
- Persons in occupational groups with exposure to blood or body fluids
- Hemodialysis patients
- Recipients of clotting factor concentrates
- Long-term international travelers
- Clients and staff of institutions for the developmentally disabled

Adapted from Weinbaum C, Williams I, Mast E, et al. Centers for Disease Control and Prevention. Recommendations for identification and public health management of persons with chronic hepatitis B virus infection. MMWR Recomm Rep 2008;57(RR-8):1–10.

---

hepatitis B vaccination for all adults who have not completed the vaccine series in settings in which a high proportion of persons are likely to be at risk for HBV infection (eg, STD/HIV testing and treatment facilities, drug-abuse treatment and prevention settings, health-care settings targeting services to intravenous-drug users (IDUs), health-care settings targeting services to MSM, and correctional facilities); (4) implement standing orders to identify adults recommended for hepatitis B vaccination and administer vaccination as part of routine services.[15]

To prevent HBV transmission, previous guidelines issued by the CDC have recommended HBsAg testing for hemodialysis patients, pregnant women, and persons known to or suspected of having been exposed to HBV (ie, infants born to HBV-infected mothers, household contacts and sex partners of infected persons, and persons with known occupational or other exposures to infectious blood or body fluids). HBsAg testing is also required for donors of blood, organs, and tissues. Testing was also recommended previously for persons born in regions with high HBV endemicity. Lastly, testing has been recommended for HIV-positive persons on the basis of their high prevalence of HBV coinfection and their increased risk for HBV-associated morbidity and mortality.[15]

Because persons with chronic HBV infections serve as the reservoir for new HBV infections in the United States, identification of these persons is needed in conjunction to vaccination strategies for elimination of HBV transmission. Therefore, the CDC recommends expanding HBV testing to include all persons born in regions with HBsAg prevalence of greater than or equal to 2%. Furthermore, HBsAg testing and vaccination are recommended for MSM and IDUs because of their increased HBsAg seroprevalence and persistent risks for acute infection. The CDC also suggests that testing should be performed in persons with alanine aminotransferase (ALT) elevations of unknown etiology and candidates for immunosuppressive therapies.[16]

Populations Recommended or Required for Routine Testing for Chronic HBV Infection

Persons born in regions of high and intermediate HBV endemicity (HBsAg prevalence ≥2%) (**Box 3**).

All persons (including immigrants, refugees, asylum seekers, and internationally adopted children) born in regions with high and intermediate endemicity of HBV infection should be tested for HBsAg, regardless of vaccination status in their country of origin.[16]

US-born persons not vaccinated as infants whose parents were born in regions with high HBV endemicity (≥8%).

If not vaccinated as infants in the United States, these persons should be tested regardless of maternal HBsAg status.[15]

Injection-drug users

First vaccine dose should be given at the same visit as that for testing for HBsAg. Testing for antibody to hepatitis B core antigen (anti-HBc) or anti-HBs should be done as well to identify susceptible persons. Susceptible persons should complete a 3-dose hepatitis B vaccine series to prevent infection from ongoing exposure.[16]

Men who have sex with men

First vaccine dose should be given at the same visit as that for testing for HBsAg. Testing for anti-HBc or anti-HBs should be done as well to identify susceptible persons. Susceptible persons should complete a 3-dose hepatitis B vaccine series to prevent infection from ongoing exposure.[16]

Box 3
Recommended or required populations for routine testing for chronic HBV

Persons born in regions of high or intermediate HBV endemicity

US-born persons not vaccinated as infants whose parents were born in regions with high HBV endemicity

MSM

Persons needing immunosuppressive therapy, including chemotherapy, immunosuppression related to organ transplantation, and immunosuppression for rheumatologic or gastroenterologic disorders

Persons with elevated ALT/AST of unknown etiology

Donors of blood, plasma, organs, tissues, or semen

Hemodialysis patients

All pregnant women

Infants born to HBsAg-positive mothers

Abbreviation: AST, aspartame aminotransferase.

Adapted from Weinbaum C, Lyerla R, Margolis HS. Centers for Disease Control and Prevention. Prevention and control of infections with hepatitis viruses in correctional settings.MMWR Recomm Rep 2003;52(RR-1):1–36.

Persons needing immunosuppressive therapy

This includes chemotherapy, immunosuppression related to organ transplantation, and immunosuppression for rheumatologic or gastroenterologic disorders.[16]

Serologic testing should test for key markers of current or prior HBV infection (HBsAg, anti-HBc, and anti-HBs). Because of elevated risk of fulminant hepatitis in chronically infected persons once suppressive therapy is initiated and risk for reactivation in persons with resolved infection, persons who are HBsAg-positive should be treated with an oral antiviral agent, and persons who are anti-HBc positive should be monitored closely for reactivation of HBV infection.[16]

Persons with elevated ALT/AST of unknown etiology

Testing for HBsAg should be performed along with other examination and laboratory testing in the context of medical evaluation.[16]

Donors of blood, plasma, organs, tissues, or semen

To prevent HBV transmission to recipients, HBsAg, anti-HBc, and HBV-DNA testing is performed.[16]

Hemodialysis patients

Serologic testing should test for markers of prior or current HBV infection (HBsAg, anti-HBc, and anti-HBs) on admission. To prevent transmission in dialysis settings, hemodialysis patients should be vaccinated against hepatitis B and revaccinated when serum anti-HBs titer falls below 10 mIU/mL. HBsAg-positive hemodialysis patients should be cohorted. Vaccine nonresponders should be tested monthly for HBsAg.[15,17]

Pregnant women

Women should be tested for HBsAg during each pregnancy, preferably in the first trimester. If an HBsAg test result is not available or if the mother was at risk for infection during pregnancy, testing should be performed at the time of admission for delivery. To prevent perinatal transmission, infants of HBsAg-positive mothers and unknown HBsAg status mothers should receive vaccination and postexposure immunoprophylaxis in accordance with recommendations within 12 hours of delivery.[15]

Infants born to HBsAg-positive mothers

Testing for HBsAg and anti-HBs should be performed in infants 1 to 2 months after completion of at least 3 doses of licensed hepatitis B vaccine series (ie, at age 9–18 months, generally at the next well-child visit) to assess the effectiveness of postexposure immunoprophylaxis. Testing should not be performed before age 9 months or within 1 month of the most recent vaccine dose. Maternal and infant medical records should be reviewed to determine whether infant received hepatitis B immune globulin (HBIG) and vaccine in accordance with recommendations.[15]

Hepatitis B Vaccines

Hepatitis B vaccines are available as a single-antigen formulation and also in fixed combination with other vaccines (**Boxes 4** and **5**). Two single-antigen vaccines are available in the United States: Recombivax HB and Engerix-B. Three licensed combination vaccines are available. Twinrix is used for vaccination of adults and contains recombinant HBsAg and inactivated HAV. Comvax is used for vaccination of infants and young children and contains recombinant HBsAg and *Haemophilus influenzae* type b polyribosylribitol phosphate conjugated to *Neisseria meningitidis* outer membrane protein complex. Pediatrix is also used for vaccination of infants and young

Box 4
Adults recommended to receive hepatitis B vaccination
Persons at risk for infection by sexual exposure
Sex partners of HBsAg-positive persons
Sexually active persons who are not in a long-term, mutually monogamous relationship (eg, persons with more than 1 sex partner during the previous 6 months
Persons seeking evaluation or treatment for an STD
MSM
Persons at risk for infection by percutaneous or mucosal exposure to blood
Current or recent injection-drug users
Household contacts of HBsAg-positive persons
Residents and staff of facilities for developmentally disabled persons
Health care and public safety workers with reasonably anticipated risk for exposure to blood or blood-contaminated body fluids
Persons with end-stage renal disease, including predialysis, hemodialysis, peritoneal dialysis, and home dialysis patients
Others
International travelers to regions with high or intermediate levels (HBsAg prevalence of $\geq 2\%$) of endemic HBV infection
Persons with chronic liver disease
Persons with HIV infection
All other persons seeking protection from HBV infection
Adapted from Mast E, Weinbaum C, Fiore A, et al. Centers for Disease Control and Prevention. A comprehensive immunization strategy to eliminate transmission of hepatitis B virus infection in the United States. MMWR Recomm Rep 2006;55(RR-16):1–23.

children and contains recombinant HBsAg, diphtheria and tetanus toxoids, and acellular pertussis adsorbed (DTaP), and inactivated poliovirus.

Hepatitis B vaccine arises from HBsAg that is purified from the plasma of persons with chronic HBV or produced by recombinant DNA technology. For vaccines in the United States, DNA technology is used to express HBsAg in yeast, which is then purified from the cells. Hepatitis B vaccines licensed in the United States are formulated to contain 10 to 40 μg of HBsAg protein/mL.[16]

Hepatitis B Immune Globulin

HBIG provides passively acquired anti-HBs and temporary protection (approximately 3–6 months) when administered in standard doses. For postexposure immunoprophylaxis, HBIG is typically given with the hepatitis B vaccine to prevent HBV infection. For those who are nonresponders to hepatitis B vaccination, HBIG administered alone is the primary means of protection after HBV exposure.[16]

Vaccination Schedule for Adults

Primary vaccination for hepatitis B consists of 3 or more IM doses administered at 0, 1, and 6 months. A protective antibody response occurs in 30% to 50% of healthy adults

---

Box 5
Settings in which hepatitis B vaccination is recommended for all adults

STD treatment facilities

HIV testing and treatment facilities

Facilities providing drug-abuse treatment and prevention services

Health care settings targeting services to injection-drug users

Correctional facilities

Health care settings targeting services to MSM

Chronic-hemodialysis facilities and end-stage renal disease programs

Institutions and nonresidential day care facilities for developmentally disabled persons

Adapted from Mast E, Weinbaum C, Fiore A, et al. Centers for Disease Control and Prevention. A comprehensive immunization strategy to eliminate transmission of hepatitis B virus infection in the United States. MMWR Recomm Rep 2006;55(RR-16):1–23.

---

40 years or younger after the first dose, 75% after the second dose, and more than 90% after the third dose. After the age of 40 years, the proportion of persons who have a protective antibody response after a 3-dose vaccination regimen declines below 90%, and by age 60 years, protective levels of antibody develop in only 75% of vaccinated persons. Other host factors, such as smoking, obesity, genetic factors, and immune suppression may contribute to decreased vaccine response. Alternative vaccination schedules at 0, 1, and 4 months or 0, 2, and 4 months have elicited dose-specific and final rates of seroprotection similar to those obtained on a 0-, 1-, and 6-month schedule.

For those aged 18 years or older with risk factors for hepatitis A and hepatitis B, the combined hepatitis A-hepatitis B vaccine (Twinrix) is indicated. This is also administered in a 3-dose schedule.[16]

Response to Vaccination

Postvaccination testing is recommended for persons whose clinical management depends on knowledge of their immune status, including certain health care and public safety workers; chronic hemodialysis patients, HIV-infected persons, and other immunocompromised persons; and sex or needle-sharing partners of HBsAg-positive persons. Among those who did not show a response to a primary 3-dose vaccine series, 25% to 50% responded to an additional vaccine dose, and 44% to 100% responded to a 3-dose revaccination series. Persons who do not have protective levels of anti-HBs 1 to 2 months after revaccination are either primary nonresponders or have unrecognized HBV infection. Genetic factors may contribute to null response to hepatitis B vaccination.[16]

Unlike immunocompetent adults, hemodialysis patients are less likely to develop protective levels of antibody as those following standard vaccination dosing; protective levels of antibody appear in only 60% to 80%.[1] Humoral response to hepatitis B vaccination is also reduced in other immunocompromised persons, such as HIV-infected persons, hematopoietic stem-cell transplant recipients, and patients undergoing chemotherapy.

Immunocompetent persons who achieve anti-HBs concentrations of greater than or equal to 10 mIU/mL after pre-exposure vaccination have nearly 100% protection against both acute disease and chronic infection, even if anti-HBs concentrations decline to less than 10 mIU/mL. Furthermore, persons who are immunocompromised and achieve and maintain a protective antibody response before exposure to HBV have a high level of protection from infection.[16]

Postexposure Prophylaxis

Following exposure to HBV, both passive-active postexposure prophylaxis with HBIG and hepatitis B vaccine and active postexposure prophylaxis using hepatitis B vaccine are highly effective in preventing infection after exposure to HBV. HBIG alone has also demonstrated effectiveness in preventing HBV transmission, but with the availability of hepatitis B vaccine, this has been used in adjunct with the vaccine. In order for postexposure prophylaxis to be effective, early administration of the initial dose of the vaccine is needed. The interval is likely 7 days or less for needlestick exposures and 14 days or less for sexual exposures.[16]

FUTURE VACCINATIONS

Worldwide, approximately 180 million people are infected with HCV. Of those infected, up to 80% develop chronic infection that frequently leads to serious liver disease such as cirrhosis and primary liver cancer. With up to 15 million people newly infected each year, there is a critical need to develop an effective vaccine.

HCV is classified into 6 distinct genotypes and more than 90 subtypes. Extensive heterogeneity is also observed within an infected individual. A significant challenge in developing a vaccine is defining protective epitopes that are recognized by antibodies conserved broadly among different HCV genotypes and subtypes. Human monoclonal antibodies have been identified that target domain B epitopes, which are frequent targets of the humoral immune response in patients with chronic hepatitis C infection. However, from a vaccine perspective, additional studies are required to determine which of the domain B epitopes may be prone to accumulate mutations under immune pressure that lead to virus escape from neutralization.[18] Furthermore, an effective vaccine will need to induce antibodies that are ideally directed at more invariant epitopes to minimize the possibility of virus escape. Therapies should consist of 2 or more antibodies recognizing different and nonoverlapping epitopes to lessen the chances of virus escape.[19]

SUMMARY

Since 1981, an HBV vaccine has been available, and for hepatitis A, since 1995. Because of the challenge in defining the protective epitopes of HCV, an effective vaccine for HCV has not yet been developed.

The ACIP recommends administration of hepatitis A vaccine for persons at increased risk, including international travelers, MSM, injection-and noninjection-drug users, and children 12 months of age or older, and catch-up vaccination for children who have not received the vaccine. The CDC also issued the following recommendations for universal hepatitis B vaccination for all adults who have not completed the vaccine series in settings in which a high proportion of persons are likely to be at risk for HBV infection (eg, STD/HIV testing and treatment facilities, drug-abuse treatment and prevention settings, health care settings targeting services to IDUs, health care settings targeting services to MSM, and correctional facilities); (4) implementation of standing orders to identify adults recommended for hepatitis B vaccination and administer vaccination as part of routine services. Testing for chronic hepatitis B should occur in those persons who have immigrated from areas of high and intermediate endemicity; those in contact with persons with chronic hepatitis B; injection-drug users; MSM; hemodialysis patients; patients who are undergoing immunosuppressive therapy; all pregnant women; patients with elevations in AST and ALT of unknown etiology; donors of blood, plasma, organs, tissues, or semen; and infants born to mothers who are HBsAg positive. Both hepatitis A and hepatitis B vaccines should also be administered to persons with chronic liver disease to prevent superinfection that may lead to hepatic decompensation. Vaccines are available as single-antigen vaccines or as combination-antigen vaccines. The recommended use of these vaccines can decrease the incidence of both hepatitis A and hepatitis B, further reducing health care costs associated with treating these acute and chronic infections.

REFERENCES

1. Centers for Disease Control and Prevention. Recommendations for identification and public health management of persons with chronic hepatitis B virus infection. MMWR Recomm Rep 2008;57(RR-8):1–20.
2. Previsani N, Lavanchy D. Hepatitis A. Switzerland: World Health Organization; 2000. p. 1–41.
3. Wasley A, Fiore A, Pell B. Hepatitis A in the era of vaccination. Epidemiol Rev 2006;28:101–11.
4. Vogt T, Wise M, Pell B, et al. Declining hepatitis A mortality in the United States during the era of hepatitis A vaccination. J Infect Dis 2008;197:1282–8.
5. Worns M, Teufel A, Kanzler A, et al. Incidence of HAV and HBV infections and vaccination rates in patients with autoimmune liver diseases. Am J Gastroenterol 2008;103(1):138–46.
6. Reiss G, Keeffe E. Review article: hepatitis vaccination in patients with chronic liver disease. Aliment Pharmacol Ther 2004;19:715–27.
7. Vento S, Garofano T, Renzini C, et al. Fulminant hepatitis associated with hepatitis A virus superinfection in patients with chronic hepatitis C. N Engl J Med 1998; 338(5):286–90.
8. Centers for Disease Control and Prevention. Prevention of hepatitis A through active or passive immunizations. MMWR Recomm Rep 1996;45(RR-15):1–23.
9. Centers for Disease Control and Prevention. Update: prevention of hepatitis A after exposure to hepatitis A virus and in international travelers. Updated recommendations of the advisory committee on immunization practices (ACIP). MMWR Recomm Rep 2007;56(41):1080–4.
10. Fiore AE, Wasley A, Bell BP, for the Advisory Committee on Immunization Practices (ACIP). Prevention of hepatitis A through active or passive immunization. MMWR Recomm Rep 2006;55(RR-07):1–23.
11. Alter M. Epidemiology of viral hepatitis and HIV co-infection. J Hepatol 2006;44: S6–9.
12. Shepard CW, Simard EP, Finelli L, et al. Hepatitis B virus infection: epidemiology and vaccination. Epidemiol Rev 2006;28:112–25.
13. Cardell K, Akerlind B, Sallberg M, et al. Excellent response rate to a double dose of the combined hepatitis A and B vaccine in previous nonresponders to hepatitis B vaccine. J Infect Dis 2008;198:299–304.
14. Centers for Disease Control and Prevention. Surveillance for acute viral hepatitis – United States, 2006. MMWR Recomm Rep 2008;57(SS-2):1–24.
15. Centers for Disease Control and Prevention. A comprehensive immunization strategy to eliminate transmission of hepatitis B virus infection in the United

States: recommendations of the advisory committee on immunization practices (ACIP): part I: immunization of infants, children, and adolescents. MMWR Recomm Rep 2005;54(RR-16):1–30.

16. Centers for Disease Control and Prevention. A comprehensive immunization strategy to eliminate transmission of hepatitis B virus infection in the United States: recommendation of the advisory committee on immunization practices (ACIP) part II: immunization of adults. MMWR Recomm Rep 2006;55(RR-16): 1–23.

17. Centers for Disease Control and Prevention. Recommendations for preventing transmission of infections among chronic hemodialysis patients. MMWR Recomm Rep 2001;50(RR-5):1–43.

18. Keck ZY, Olson O, Gal-Tanamy M, et al. A point mutation leading to hepatitis C virus escape from neutralization by a monoclonal antibody to a conserved conformational epitope. J Virol 2008;82:6067–72.

19. Perotti M, Mancini N, Diotti R, et al. Identification of a broadly cross-reacting and neutralizing human monoclonal antibody directed against the hepatitis C virus e2 protein. J Virol 2008;82:1047–52.

Care of the Cirrhotic Patient

Priya Grewal, MD[a],*, Paul Martin, MD[b]

KEYWORDS

- Cirrhosis • Complications • Ascites
- Encephalopathy • HCC

Anticipation and management of complications in a patient with cirrhosis are key aspects for a patient who may ultimately require liver transplantation. Timely surveillance for varices and hepatocellular carcinoma (HCC), prophylaxis against spontaneous bacterial peritonitis (SBP), and early diagnosis of minimal or overt hepatic encephalopathy (HE) can delay life-threatening complications, reduce need for hospitalization, and potentially improve survival pending liver transplantation. A patient with well-compensated cirrhosis has a 5-year survival rate of 90% and a good likelihood of living 10 years without decompensation.[1] With the onset of decompensation, in the form of ascites, variceal bleeding, or HE, the survival rate decreases to less than 50% at 5 years, and these events should prompt referral of the patient for liver transplantation.

VARICEAL SCREENING AND MANAGEMENT

When cirrhosis is first diagnosed, varices are present in 30% to 40% of patients with well-compensated cirrhosis and in 60% of those with overt decompensation.[2–4] A study[5] in 2006 suggests that the appearance of varices in patients with compensated cirrhosis indicates a change from a clinical stage with a very low risk of death at 1 year (stage 1, 1% risk) to an intermediate risk stage (stage 2, 3.4% risk). The occurrence of variceal bleeding heralds the progression to decompensation of liver disease and portends a very high risk of death (stage 4, 57% risk of death at 1 year). The current consensus is that every cirrhotic patient should be endoscopically screened for varices at the time of diagnosis.[6] The aim of the screening for esophageal varices is to define patients who would benefit from prophylactic treatment to prevent variceal bleeding.

In patients without varices on initial endoscopy, it is recommended that endoscopy should be repeated after 2 to 3 years. The expected progression to moderate/large varices and subsequent variceal bleeding in these patients is less than 10% at

[a] Division of Liver Diseases, Recanati/Miller Transplantation Institute, The Mount Sinai Medical Center, One Gustave L. Levy Place, Box 1104, New York, NY 10029, USA
[b] Division of Hepatology, Schiff Liver Institute/Center for Liver Diseases, University of Miami Miller School of Medicine, 1500 NW 12 Avenue, Jackson Medical Tower, E-1101, Miami, FL 33136, USA
* Corresponding author.
E-mail address: priya.grewal@mountsinai.org (P. Grewal).

Clin Liver Dis 13 (2009) 331–340
doi:10.1016/j.cld.2009.02.006
1089-3261/09/$ – see front matter © 2009 Elsevier Inc. All rights reserved.

liver.theclinics.com

3 years.[7,8] On the other hand, in patients with small varices on initial endoscopy and an expected progression of variceal size by 10% to 15% per year, endoscopy should be repeated every 2 years. In patients with advanced cirrhosis or red wale marks, a 6-month to 1-year interval should be recommended.[7,8] In this group of patients, the risk of imminent bleeding is very high.

Recently, the endoscopic videocapsule has been suggested as a less-invasive alternative to endoscopy for variceal screening. Once swallowed, the videocapsule records images at predetermined intervals. In the 2 published studies, capsule endoscopy allowed a correct identification of esophageal varices in 80% of cases.[9,10] In one study, capsule endoscopy accurately assessed red wale marks.[9] However, it had poor accuracy in assessing variceal size or in identifying the presence of hypertensive gastropathy or gastric varices.[11]

Prevention of the First Bleeding Episode

Beta-adrenergic blocking agents (β-blockers) are currently not recommended to prevent the initial development of esophageal varices. A recent study randomized 213 patients with cirrhosis and portal hypertension without varices on screening endoscopy to receive timolol (a nonselective β-blocker) or placebo for a median of 55 months.[2] The primary end point was development of esophageal varices or variceal hemorrhage. The secondary end points were the onset of ascites, encephalopathy, liver transplantation, or death. There was no difference in any end point between the 2 treatment groups (intention-to-treat analysis). Adverse events were more frequent in the timolol group.

In the past, only patients with medium to large varices were considered for prophylactic measures to prevent variceal bleeding with β-blockers, whereas the beneficial effects of β-blockers were less established in patients with small varices.[12] However, in the recent Baveno IV consensus conference, it was proposed that an accurate distinction of small from large varices was difficult.[6] On the other hand, it is well established that small varices with red signs or, in patients with Child-Pugh class C cirrhosis, bleeding risk are similar to that of big varices.[13] A study also showed that β-blockers may reduce the rate of progression from small to large varices and decrease the incidence of variceal bleeding in patients with small varices.[14] Therefore, the current recommendation is to extend prophylactic treatment to patients with small varices with red signs or Child-Pugh C.[6]

Endoscopic band ligation (EBL) is effective in preventing the initial variceal bleeding in patients with medium to large varices.[15] Sixteen trials have compared EBL with β-blockers as a first-line option for primary prophylaxis of variceal bleeding.[16–31] A meta-analysis of these trials showed an advantage of EBL over β-blockers in terms of prevention of first bleeding, without differences in mortality, although 6 of these trials are available only in abstract form. When the meta-analysis is restricted to published studies, there is no significant benefit from EBL compared to β-blockers. The recommendation made at the 2005 Baveno consensus conference is that nonselective β-blockers should be considered as first-choice treatment to prevent first variceal bleeding, whereas EBL should be offered to patients with medium/large varices who have contraindications or intolerance to β-blockers.[6] Increased bleeding in patients with large varices or red wale signs who have undergone primary EBL has been reported in a recent study. In this trial, EBL was compared with no treatment in patients with contraindications to β-blockers. The trial was stopped prematurely due to a high rate (12%) of iatrogenic bleeding in the band ligation group.[32]

A study was conducted to determine the accurate interval between EBL sessions with emphasis on improved effectiveness and reduced complications of EBL. EBL was performed every 2 weeks compared to every 2 months. This trial included patients with and without previous bleeding, though most patients underwent EBL as primary prophylaxis.[33] The 2-month-interval, EBL regimen obtained a higher total eradication rate and a lower recurrence rate. No patient in either group developed variceal bleeding. Thus, current evidence favors a less frequent interval. After successful eradication, follow-up endoscopy should be performed every 6 months, and varices should be eradicated upon recurrence.

HCC SCREENING

HCC screening is recommended in cirrhotic patients. It is also recommended in Hepatitis B carriers (HBsAg positive) even without overt cirrhosis, especially those with a family history of HCC, infected individuals from Africa older than 20 years, and Asian males and females older than 40 and 50 years, respectively. Current evidence supports screening in patients with cirrhosis from hepatitis C, alcohol, genetic hemochromatosis, and primary biliary cirrhosis and possibly in patients with alpha 1-antitrypsin deficiency, nonalcoholic steatohepatitis, and autoimmune hepatitis.[34]

In a randomized, controlled trial in China of nearly 19,000 HBV-infected patients, HCC surveillance was performed with testing of serum alpha-fetoprotein (AFP) and abdominal ultrasound (US) at 6-month intervals. The study showed improved survival, with a 37% reduction in HCC-related mortality.[35,36] Other observational studies have shown survival benefit with surveillance when HCC was diagnosed early and curative treatments were applied. The most widely used tools for HCC surveillance are AFP and liver US. Based on the estimated HCC doubling time, the recommended surveillance interval is 6 months, although a 1-year interval may be equally effective.[37]

Recent studies generally indicate 60% sensitivity and 90% specificity for liver US.[38] A serum AFP level of 20 ng/mL commonly used as the upper limit of normal has low sensitivity (25%–65%) for detecting HCC. Patients with chronic liver disease, especially those with a high degree of hepatocyte regeneration (as in hepatitis C virus [HCV]), can have elevated serum AFP in the absence of malignancy.[39] In patients undergoing HCC surveillance, while awaiting liver transplantation, computed tomography (CT) is associated with the greatest gain in life expectancy and is possibly cost-effective in this setting.[40]

Once a screening test is abnormal or there is a clinical suspicion that a patient may have HCC, appropriate imaging is very important for the diagnosis and staging of this tumor. The most reliable diagnostic tests are triple-phase, helical CT and triple-phase, dynamic, contrast-enhanced magnetic resonance imaging (MRI).[41,42] HCC derives its blood supply predominantly from the hepatic artery, whereas the remainder of the nontumorous liver receives both arterial and portal blood. The hallmark of HCC on CT scan or MRI is the presence of arterial enhancement followed by delayed hypointensity of the tumor, with washout in the portal venous and delayed phases.[43] The presence of arterial enhancement followed by washout has a sensitivity and specificity of 90% and 95%, respectively. Though 71% of patients with HCC will have arterial enhancement and washout on more than 1 test, the reminder do not have these features and, therefore, may require additional tests for the diagnosis of HCC. Currently, serum AFP levels more than 200 ng/mL are highly specific for HCC in patients with cirrhosis and coinciding radiologic evidence of focal hepatic lesions.[35] However, the sensitivity of AFP is much lower, because it has been reported that only one-third of patients with HCC have AFP levels higher than 100 ng/mL.

ASCITES: DIAGNOSIS AND MANAGEMENT

Ascites is the most common complication of cirrhosis. After its onset, the expected 2-year survival rate is 50%, so cirrhotic patients who develop ascites should be considered for transplant.[44] A diagnostic paracentesis should be performed in all patients with recent-onset ascites.

This is to confirm that the serum-ascites albumin gradient value is at least 1.1 g/dL, which is diagnostic of ascites related to portal hypertension.[45] A white cell count should also be done to exclude SBP, which is incidentally discovered in 10% to 25% of hospitalized cirrhotic patients. Patients should be encouraged to stay on a 2-gram, sodium-restricted diet but the restriction should not be so stringent that it compromises their nutritional status. Fluid restriction is recommended at a serum sodium less than 120 to 125 mmol/L, although most cirrhotic patients have symptoms only at serum sodium levels less than 110 mmol/L.[46] Mild to moderate ascites is controlled best by the combined diuretic regimen of spironolactone (100 mg) and furosemide (40 mg), taken in single doses in the morning.[47] The doses of both diuretics can be increased simultaneously every 3 to 5 days, maintaining the 100:40 ratio to preserve normokalemia, if weight loss is not adequate (1–2 lbs/day). This approach of salt restriction and diuretic is effective in 90% of patients. Diuretics should be held if patients develop encephalopathy, serum sodium less than 120 mmol/L, or serum creatinine that rises above "normal."[47] Serum creatinine level in advanced cirrhosis may underestimate renal dysfunction because of reduced muscle mass, the substrate for creatinine production. Approximately 10% of cirrhotic patients ultimately develop refractory ascites. These patients may require large-volume paracentesis periodically or be considered for a more definitive intervention, such as a transjugular intrahepatic portosystemic shunt or liver transplantation.

Spontaneous Bacterial Peritonitis

SBP is a spontaneous infection of the ascitic fluid, which usually develops in patients with clinically obvious ascites or advanced liver disease. A polymorphonuclear leukocyte cell count greater than 250/mm^3 on ascitic tap confirms the diagnosis of SBP.

Secondary Prophylaxis

After a single bout of SBP, there is a 70% 1-year cumulative probability of developing a subsequent episode of SBP, and prophylaxis is recommended.[48] Oral norfloxacin (400 mg/d) or ciprofloxacin (750 mg once every week) can reduce the risk for SBP to 20%.[49]

Primary Prophylaxis

In cirrhotic ascites, a total protein content less than 1 g/dL,[50] serum bilirubin level greater than 3.2 mg/dL, and platelet count less than 98,000/mm^3 predicted an approximate risk of 55% for developing SBP within the next year.[51] SBP prophylaxis is appropriate in this setting as supported by 2 recent studies.[52,53] In the first study, 68 patients with either advanced liver failure and low protein ascites with a Child-Pugh score more than 9 or impaired renal function and hyponatremia were randomized to receive norfloxacin 400 mg/d or placebo for 1 year. This resulted in a statistically significant reduction in the probability of developing SBP and hepatic renal syndrome. The improved 3-month and 1-year survival was surprisingly related to a decrease in the incidence of hepatic renal syndrome in the treated group. The high prevalence of alcoholic cirrhosis and active alcohol use (20%–25%) in both groups may, however, have confounded the results.[52] In the second study, 100 cirrhotic patients with low ascitic protein (<1.5 mg/dL) were randomized to Ciprofloxacin 500 mg/d versus placebo for 12 months. At 1 year, the incidence of SBP was 4 times lower in patients in the treated group who also had a significantly better survival, (P<.04).[53] Based on the high 30-day mortality with a bout of SBP (20%–30%), which has improved with earlier diagnosis, treatment, and use of albumin in the recent years, primary prophylaxis should be initiated in all high-risk patients.

MINIMAL HEPATIC ENCEPHALOPATHY

HE is a myriad neuropsychiatric abnormalities seen in 50% to 70% patients with cirrhosis.[54] Patients with HE have impaired intellectual functioning, personality changes, altered level of consciousness, and neuromuscular dysfunction. Although patients with overt HE are usually diagnosed clinically and treated with lactulose and rifaximin, the awareness of mild HE or minimal HE (MHE) is still evolving. There are no recognizable clinical symptoms of MHE, but patients do have mild cognitive and psychomotor deficits. In the absence of a gold standard for determining MHE, neuropsychological and neurophysiologic methods have been the most trusted and widely used tests to diagnose this condition. The Inhibitory Control Test (ICT) is a computerized test of attention and response inhibition that has been used to characterize attention-deficit disorder, schizophrenia, and traumatic brain injury. ICT has also been validated for the diagnosis of MHE.[55] MHE is considered clinically relevant for several reasons. Besides impairing patients' daily functioning and health-related quality of life (HRQOL), MHE may render many patients unfit to drive a car.[56] It also predicts the development of overt HE and is associated with a poor prognosis.[57,58] The pathogenesis of MHE is believed to be similar to that of overt HE.

A recent study[59] evaluated the role of lactulose in 61 patients with MHE. Patients were treated with lactulose or given no treatment for 3 months. Both cognitive function and HRQOL were significantly improved in the group treated with lactulose. The role of probiotic yogurt was studied in 25 patients with MHE assigned to yogurt versus no treatment in a 2:1 ratio. In the treated group, 71% reversed their MHE, and no subject developed overt HE compared to the control group.[60]

The diagnosis of MHE remains time consuming, although it clearly affects the QOL of patients with cirrhosis and is a risk factor for mortality related to accidents. Treatment modalities appear to be promising and are similar to the ones used in overt HE.

IMMUNIZATION

Patients who have advanced cirrhosis have increased morbidity and mortality associated with viral and bacterial infections.[61,62] The Advisory Committee on Immunization Practices recommends that all patients who have chronic liver disease be vaccinated against hepatitis A virus (HAV), hepatitis B virus (HBV), pneumococcus, and influenza. Patients with chronic HBV who contract acute HAV have a more severe clinical course and higher death rate, especially older patients who have cirrhosis, based on epidemiologic data from the Centers for Disease Control and Prevention and large studies in Shanghai, Japan, and Greece.[63–66]

Similar results were noted for HAV superinfection in 432 patients who had HCV during a 7-year period. Seven of 17 patients with acute HAV had fulminant hepatitis, and 6 died.[67] Acute HBV superimposed on chronic HCV has also been implicated as a cause of fulminant hepatitis.[68]

Response to the pneumococcal vaccine tends to decline by 6 months after inoculation in cirrhotic patients and continues to decrease after transplantation, although antibody titers remain higher than prevaccination levels.[69] Efforts should be made to improve adherence to these recommendations, as only 55% and 34% of patients who have chronic liver disease are immunized against influenza and pneumococcus, respectively.[70]

The rate of anti-HAV seropositivity from prior resolved infection in patients who have chronic liver disease is approximately 55% in the United States and 30% in the general population, with increasing prevalence in older patients.[71] Based on this, a selective strategy of vaccination against HAV is used in patients who have chronic liver disease (ie, checking serology before vaccine administration). It should be given as early as possible in patients who have chronic liver disease, as the response rate after the booster dose varies from 98% in early cirrhotic patients to 65% in decompensated cirrhotic patients awaiting transplantation.[72,73]

Hepatitis B vaccination is recommended in patients who have chronic HCV infection if they are HBV naive with absent HBV total core and surface antibody. The response rate varies from more than 95% in mild to moderate liver disease to only 30% to 50% in patients who have decompensated cirrhosis.[74] A strategy of using double dose (40 mg) and an accelerated schedule (0, 1, and 2 months) increases seroconversion rates to between 44% and 62%.[75]

SUMMARY

Patients with well-compensated cirrhosis can expect at least several years before they develop complications that may affect their overall survival. Early detection and prompt management of many of these complications may delay the need for liver transplantation at least temporarily and decrease mortality.

REFERENCES

1. Fattovich G, Giustina G, Degos F, et al. Morbidity and mortality in compensated cirrhosis type C: a retrospective follow-up study of 384 patients. Gastroenterology 1997;112:463–72.
2. Groszmann RJ, Garcia-Tsao G, Bosch J, et al. Beta blockers to prevent gastro-esophageal varices in patients with cirrhosis. N Engl J Med 2005;353:2254–61.
3. D'Amico G, Pagliaro L, Bosch J. The treatment of portal hypertension: a meta-analytic review. Hepatology 1995;22:332–54.
4. D'Amico G, Luca A. Natural history—clinical-haemodynamic correlations: prediction of the risk of bleeding. Baillieres Clin Gastroenterol 1997;11:243–56.
5. D'Amico G, Garcia-Tsao G, Pagliaro L. Natural history and prognostic indicators of survival in cirrhosis: a systematic review of 118 studies. J Hepatol 2006;44: 217–31.
6. de Franchis R. Evolving consensus in portal hypertension: report of the Baveno IV consensus workshop on methodology of diagnosis and therapy in portal hypertension. J Hepatol 2005;43:167–76.
7. Merli M, Nicolini G, Angeloni S, et al. Incidence and natural history of small esophageal varices in cirrhotic patients. J Hepatol 2003;38:266–72.
8. de Franchis R. Evaluation and follow-up of patients with cirrhosis and oesophageal varices. J Hepatol 2003;38:361–3.
9. Eisen GM, Eliakim R, Zaman A, et al. The accuracy of PillCam ESO capsule endoscopy versus conventional upper endoscopy for the diagnosis of esophageal varices: a prospective three-center pilot study. Endoscopy 2006;38:31–5.

10. Lapalus MG, Dumortier J, Fumex F, et al. Esophageal capsule endoscopy versus esophagogastroduodenoscopy for evaluating portal hypertension: a prospective comparative study of performance and tolerance. Endoscopy 2006;38:36–41.

11. Frenette C, Kuldau JG, Hillebrand D, et al. Comparison of esophageal pill endoscopy and conventional endoscopy for variceal screening. Hepatology 2006; 44(Suppl 1):445A.

12. D'Amico G, Pagliaro L, Bosch J. Pharmacological treatment of portal hypertension: an evidence-based approach. Semin Liver Dis 1999;19:475–505.

13. North Italian Endoscopic Club. Prediction of the first variceal hemorrhage in patients with cirrhosis of the liver and esophageal varices: a prospective multicenter study. The North Italian Endoscopic Club for the study and treatment of Esophageal Varices. N Engl J Med 1988;319:983–9.

14. Merkel C, Marin R, Angeli P, et al. A placebo-controlled clinical trial of nadolol in the prophylaxis of growth of small esophageal varices in cirrhosis. Gastroenterology 2004;127:476–84.

15. Imperiale TF, Chalasani N. A meta-analysis of endoscopic variceal ligation for primary prophylaxis of esophageal variceal bleeding. Hepatology 2001;33: 802–7.

16. Lo GH, Chen WC, Chen MH, et al. Endoscopic ligation vs. nadolol in the prevention of first variceal bleeding in patients with cirrhosis. Gastrointest Endosc 2004; 59:333–8.

17. Chen CY, Sheu MZ, Tsai TL, et al. Endoscopic variceal ligation with multiple band ligator for prophylaxis of first hemorrhage esophageal varices. Endoscopy 1999; 31(Suppl 1):35A.

18. Schepke M, Kleber G, Nurnberg D, et al. Ligation versus propranolol for the primary prophylaxis of variceal bleeding in cirrhosis. Hepatology 2004;40: 65–72.

19. Song H, Shin JW, Kim HI, et al. A prospective randomized trial between the prophylactic endoscopic variceal ligation and propranolol administration for prevention of first bleeding in cirrhotic patients with high-risk esophageal varices. J Hepatol 2000;32(Suppl 2):41A.

20. Sarin SK, Lamba GS, Kumar M, et al. Comparison of endoscopic ligation and propranolol for the primary prevention of variceal bleeding. N Engl J Med 1999;340:988–93.

21. de la Mora G, Farca-Belsaguy AA, Uribe M, et al. Ligation vs propranolol for primary prophylaxis of variceal bleeding using multiple band ligator and objective measurements of treatment adequacy: preliminary results. Gastroenterology 2000;118:6511A.

22. Lui HF, Stanley AJ, Forrest EH, et al. Primary prophylaxis of variceal hemorrhage: a randomized controlled trial comparing band ligation, propranolol, and isosorbide mononitrate. Gastroenterology 2002;123:735–44.

23. Jutabha R, Jensen DM, Martin P, et al. Randomized study comparing banding and propranolol to prevent initial variceal hemorrhage in cirrhotics with high-risk esophageal varices. Gastroenterology 2005;128:870–81.

24. Thuluvath PJ, Maheshwari A, Jagannath S, et al. A randomized controlled trial of beta-blockers versus endoscopic band ligation for primary prophylaxis: a large sample size is required to show a difference in bleeding rates. Dig Dis Sci 2005;50:407–10.

25. De BK, Ghoshal UC, Das T, et al. Endoscopic variceal ligation for primary prophylaxis of oesophageal variceal bleed: preliminary report of a randomized controlled trial. J Gastroenterol Hepatol 1999;14:220–4.

26. Drastich P, Lata J, Petrtyl J, et al. Endoscopic variceal band ligation in comparison with propranolol in prophylaxis of first variceal bleeding in patients with liver cirrhosis. J Hepatol 2005;42:202A.

27. Lay CS, Tsai YT, Lee FY, et al. Endoscopic variceal ligation versus propranolol in prophylaxis of first variceal bleeding in patients with cirrhosis. J Gastroenterol Hepatol 2006;21:413–9.

28. Psilopoulos D, Galanis P, Goulas S, et al. Endoscopic variceal ligation vs. propranolol for prevention of first variceal bleeding: a randomized controlled trial. Eur J Gastroenterol Hepatol 2005;17:1111–7.

29. Abdelfattah MH, Rashed MA, Elfakhry AA, et al. Endoscopic variceal ligation versus pharmacological treatment for primary prophylaxis of variceal bleeding: a randomized study. J Hepatol 2006;44(Suppl 2):83A.

30. Gheorghe C, Gheorghe L, Vadan R, et al. Prophylactic banding ligation of high-risk esophageal varices in patients on the waiting list for liver transplantation: an interim analysis. J Hepatol 2002;36(Suppl 1):38A.

31. Norberto L, Polese L, Cillo U, et al. A randomized study comparing ligation with propranolol for primary prophylaxis of variceal bleeding in candidates for liver transplantation. Liver Transpl 2007;13:1272–8.

32. Triantos C, Vlachogiannakos J, Armonis A, et al. Primary prophylaxis of variceal bleeding in cirrhotics unable to take beta-blockers: a randomized trial of ligation. Aliment Pharmacol Ther 2005;21:1435–43.

33. Yoshida H, Mamada Y, Taniai N, et al. A randomized control trial of bi-monthly versus bi-weekly endoscopic variceal ligation of esophageal varices. Am J Gastroenterol 2005;100:2005–9.

34. El-Serag, Marrero J, Rudolph L, et al. Diagnosis and treatment of Hepatocellular Carcinoma. Gastroenterology 2008;134:1752–63.

35. Bruix J, Sherman M. Management of hepatocellular carcinoma. Hepatology 2005; 42:1208–36.

36. Zhang BH, Yang BH, Tang ZY. Randomized controlled trial of screening for hepatocellular carcinoma. J Cancer Res Clin Oncol 2004;130:417–22.

37. Trevisani F, De NS, Rapaccini G, et al. Semiannual and annual surveillance of cirrhotic patients for hepatocellular carcinoma: effects on cancer stage and patient survival (Italian experience). Am J Gastroenterol 2002;97:734–44.

38. Bolondi L, Sofia S, Siringo S, et al. Surveillance programme of cirrhotic patients for early diagnosis and treatment of hepatocellular carcinoma: a cost effectiveness analysis. Gut 2001;48:251–9.

39. Bayati N, Silverman AL, Gordon SC. Serum alpha-fetoprotein levels and liver histology in patients with chronic hepatitis C. Am J Gastroenterol 1998;93: 2452–6.

40. Saab S, Ly D, Nieto J, et al. Hepatocellular carcinoma screening in patients waiting for liver transplantation: a decision analytic model. Liver Transpl 2003;9:672–81.

41. Choi D, Kim SH, Lim JH, et al. Detection of hepatocellular carcinoma: combined T2-weighted and dynamic gadolinium-enhanced MRI versus combined CT during arterial portography and CT hepatic arteriography. J Comput Assist Tomogr 2001;25:777–85.

42. Arguedas MR, Chen VK, Eloubeidi MA, et al. Screening for hepatocellular carcinoma in patients with hepatitis C cirrhosis: a cost-utility analysis. Am J Gastroenterol 2003;98:679–90.

43. Marrero JA, Hussain HK, Nghiem HV, et al. Improving the prediction of hepatocellular carcinoma in cirrhotic patients with an arterially enhancing liver mass. Liver Transpl 2005;11:281–9.

44. D'Amico G, Morabito A, Pagliaro L, et al. Survival and prognostic indicators in compensated and decompensated cirrhosis. Dig Dis Sci 1986;31:468–75.
45. Runyon BA, Montano AA, Akriviadis EA, et al. The serum-ascites albumin gradient is superior to the exudate-transudate concept in the differential diagnosis of ascites. Ann Intern Med 1992;117:215–20.
46. Runyon BA. Management of the adult patient with ascites due to cirrhosis. Hepatology 2004;39:841–56.
47. Runyon BA. Care of patients with ascites. N Engl J Med 1994;330:337–42.
48. Tito L, Rimola A, Gines P, et al. Recurrence of spontaneous bacterial peritonitis in cirrhosis: frequency and predictive factors. Hepatology 1988;8:27–31.
49. Gines P, Rimola A, Planas R, et al. Norfloxacin prevents spontaneous bacterial peritonitis recurrence in cirrhosis: results of a double-blind, placebo-controlled trial. Hepatology 1990;12:716–24.
50. Llach J, Rimola A, Navasa M, et al. Incidence and predictive factors of first episode of spontaneous bacterial peritonitis in cirrhosis with ascites: relevance of ascitic fluid protein concentration. Hepatology 1992;16:724–7.
51. Guarner C, Sola R, Soriano G, et al. Risk of a first community-acquired spontaneous bacterial peritonitis in cirrhotics with low ascitic fluid protein levels. Gastroenterology 1999;117:495–9.
52. Fernandez J, Navasa M, Planas R, et al. Primary prophylaxis of spontaneous bacterial peritonitis delays hepatorenal syndrome and improves survival in cirrhosis. Gastroenterology 2007;133:818–24.
53. Terg R, Fassio E, Guevara M, et al. Ciprofloxacin in primary prophylaxis of spontaneous bacterial peritonitis: a randomized, placebo-controlled study. J Hepatol 2008;48:774–9.
54. Riordan SM, Williams R. Treatment of Hepatic encephalopathy. N Engl J Med 1997;337:473–9.
55. Bajaj J, Hafeezullah M, Franco J, et al. Inhibitory Control Test for the Diagnosis of Minimal Hepatic Encephalopathy. Gastroenterology 2008;135(5): 1591–600.e1.
56. Wein C, Koch H, Popp B, et al. Minimal hepatic encephalopathy impairs fitness to drive. Hepatology 2004;39:739–45.
57. Romero-Gomez M, Boza F, Garcia-Valdecasas MS, et al. Subclinical hepatic encephalopathy predicts the development of overt hepatic encephalopathy. Am J Gastroenterol 2001;96:2718–23.
58. Amodio P, Del Piccolo F, Marchetti P, et al. Clinical features and survival of cirrhotic patients with subclinical cognitive alterations detected by the number connection test and computerized psychometric tests. Hepatology 1999;29: 1662–7.
59. Prasad S, Dhiman R, Duseja A, et al. Lactulose improves cognitive functions and health- related quality of patients with cirrhosis who have minimal hepatic encephalopathy. Hepatology 2007;45:549–59.
60. Bajaj JS, Saejan K, Christensen KM, et al. Probiotic yogurt for treatment of minimal hepatic encephalopathy. Am J Gastroenterol 2008;103(7):1707–15.
61. Navasa M, Rimola A, Rodé s J. Bacterial infections in liver disease. Semin Liver Dis 1997;17:323–33.
62. Duchini A, Viernes ME, Nyberg LM, et al. Hepatic decompensation in patients with cirrhosis during infection with influenza A. Arch Intern Med 2000;160: 113–5.
63. Keeffe EB. Is hepatitis A more severe in patients with chronic hepatitis B and other chronic liver diseases? Am J Gastroenterol 1995;90:201–5.

64. Yao G. Clinical spectrum and natural history of viral hepatitis in a 1988 Shanghai epidemic. In: Hollinger FB, Lemon SM, Margolis H, editors. Viral hepatitis and liver disease. Baltimore (MD): Lippincott Williams & Wilkins; 1991. p. 76–8.

65. Fukumoto Y, Okita K, Konishi T, et al. Hepatitis A infection in chronic carriers of hepatitis B virus. In: Sung J-L, Chen D-S, editors. Viral hepatitis and hepatocellular carcinoma. Amsterdam: Excerpta Medica; 1990. p. 43–8.

66. Papachristou AA, Dumas AS, Katsouyannopoulos VC. Dissociation of alanine aminotransferase values in acute hepatitis A patients with and without past experience to the hepatitis B virus. Epidemiol Infect 1991;106:397–402.

67. Vento S, Garofano T, Renzini C, et al. Fulminant hepatitis associated with hepatitis A superinfection in patients with chronic hepatitis C. N Engl J Med 1998;338:286–90.

68. Fé ray C, Gigou M, Samuel D, et al. Hepatitis C virus RNA and hepatitis B virus DNA in serum and liver of patients with fulminant hepatitis. Gastroenterology 1993;104:549–55.

69. McCashland TM, Preheim LC, Gentry MJ. Pneumococcal vaccine response in cirrhosis and liver transplantation. J Infect Dis 2000;181:757–60.

70. Arguedas MR, McGuire BM, Fallon MB. Implementation of vaccination in patients with cirrhosis. Dig Dis Sci 2002;47:384–7.

71. Saab S, Lee C, Shpaner A, et al. Seroepidemiology of hepatitis A in patients with chronic liver disease. J Viral Hepat 2005;12:101–5.

72. Arguedas MR, Johnson A, Eloubeidi MA, et al. Immunogenicity of hepatitis A vaccination in decompensated cirrhotic patients. Hepatology 2001;34:28–31.

73. Smallwood GA, Coloura CT, Martinez E, et al. Can patients awaiting liver transplantation elicit an immune response to the hepatitis A vaccine? Transplant Proc 2002;34:3289–90.

74. Dominguez M, Barcena R, Garcia M, et al. Vaccination against hepatitis B virus in cirrhotic patients on liver transplant waiting list. Liver Transpl 2000;6:440–2.

75. Arslan M, Wiesner RH, Sievers C, et al. Double-dose accelerated hepatitis B vaccine in patients with end-stage liver disease. Liver Transpl 2001;7:314–20.

Index

Note: Page numbers of article titles are in **boldface** type.

Clin Liver Dis 13 (2009) 341–350
doi:10.1016/S1089-3261(09)00022-1
1089-3261/09/$ – see front matter © 2009 Elsevier Inc. All rights reserved.

liver.theclinics.com

Moving?

Make sure your subscription moves with you!

To notify us of your new address, find your **Clinics Account Number** (located on your mailing label above your name), and contact customer service at:

E-mail: elspcs@elsevier.com

800-654-2452 (subscribers in the U.S. & Canada)
314-453-7041 (subscribers outside of the U.S. & Canada)

Fax number: 314-523-5170

Elsevier Periodicals Customer Service
11830 Westline Industrial Drive
St. Louis, MO 63146

*To ensure uninterrupted delivery of your subscription, please notify us at least 4 weeks in advance of move.

Printed and bound by CPI Group (UK) Ltd, Croydon, CR0 4YY

03/10/2024

01040445-0017